Integrating CBT with Experiential Theory and Practice

This workbook elucidates the techniques clinicians will encounter using the cognitive experiential (psychodrama) group therapy (CEGT) model.

This model incorporates cognitive behavioral and psychodramatic interventions to help identify and modify negative thinking, behavior, and interpersonal patterns. Beginning with a brief overview of cognitive behavioral therapy (CBT) and psychodrama, the book highlights concepts and techniques that are most relevant to CEGT session content. The second half of the workbook provides a description of CEGT and what group members should expect through their engagement in this therapy. Featured throughout are tables and exercises that create pathways to challenge dysfunctional thinking along with blank worksheets to be used by group members located in the appendices.

Readers will learn techniques to challenge negative thought patterns and increase engagement in positive and success-based experiences through clear guidelines for behavioral interventions to help move individuals from negativity to a more positive life space.

Thomas W. Treadwell, EdD, is a professor of psychology at West Chester University, clinical associate at the Center for Cognitive Therapy at the Perelman School of Medicine at the University of Pennsylvania, and editor for *The Group Psychologist*, Division 49, Society of Group Psychology and Group Psychotherapy, American Psychological Association.

"This text is innovative and essential for readers looking to incorporate cognitive therapy and psychodrama elements in group treatment. Treadwell's approach emphasizes humanism, creativity, and positivity in the therapeutic environment. The concise descriptions, case formulations and worksheets will be useful to any mental health professional!"

Aaron T. Beck, MD, professor emeritus of Psychiatry,
University of Pennsylvania

"This workbook provides in depth look at an innovative approach to group therapy, one in which the powerful role-playing processes of psychodrama are coupled with the insight building tools of cognitive behavior therapy to create a positive, healing group process where individual change can take place. *Integrating CBT with Experiential Theory and Practice* is a brilliant volume jam packed with exceptional tools and acuity. This is a powerful guide for both beginner and experienced clinicians alike."

Jonathan D. Moreno, PhD, David and Lyn Silfen
professor, University of Pennsylvania

"Integrative models produce the highest levels of patient improvement in the small group treatment literature. Strategic integration of two or more efficacious group treatments within a single protocol has proven to be uniquely efficacious treatment for difficult patient populations that present with a complex multi-faceted clinical profile. Treadwell begins with the most efficacious group protocol—cognitive behavioral therapy—and merges it with one of its most engaging—experiential. Integrating CBT with Experiential Theory and Practice begins with an excellent summary of these two well-known group treatments. It then carefully lays out how to integrate key components of each model illustrating case conceptualization and in-session techniques. The reader is provided with clear clinical examples on how to apply the model with both adult and adolescent clients and the worksheets bring to life core treatment components of CBT and psychodrama. A particular strength is application of the Cognitive Experiential Group Therapy (CEGT) model for adolescents and individuals with social anxiety disorder along with expanded appendices filled with worksheets. The model contains empirically supported interventions but has ample flexibility to accommodate varied clinical conditions. I look forward to future research testing the effects of another integrative group model."

Gary Burlingame, PhD, CGP, DFAGPA, professor and chair of
Psychology, Brigham Young University

"*Integrating CBT with Experiential Theory and Practice: A Group Therapy Workbook* is true to title and contains large amounts of useful information for those interested in knowing more about these topics. This text is tight and concise, yet abundant with the basic information necessary to wrap your head around the implementation and leadership of cognitive behavioral therapy. This book is a kit that gives you solid understanding of a range of topics that together form the core of a cognitive experiential orientation and group interventions using Moreno's theories and techniques. There is a lot of wisdom in these chapters and it is presented in a useful and informative voice that many readers will find both encouraging and easily understandable."

Joshua M. Gross, PhD, ABPP, CGP, director
of Group Programs, Florida State University

"Thomas Treadwell et al have assembled a very helpful group therapy workbook combining the skills of Cognitive Behavioral Therapy (CBT) and Experiential (Psychodramatic) Theory (PT) to create Cognitive Psychodrama Group Therapy (CEGT). The handbook is a solid presentation of Cognitive Behavioral Therapy, systematically described in sections related to schemas, core beliefs, cognitive distortions, intermediate beliefs, and automatic thoughts. Graduate students and group members alike will be able to review clear information about CBT and Psychodramatic Therapy, with focus on the latter simply because there is less available in the extant literature regarding the powerful action-oriented psychodrama techniques pioneered by Moreno over sixty years ago. Useful session-by-session outlines are punctuated by glossaries, role-plays, worksheets and charts. Treadwell is an expert at application."

Sally H. Barlow, PhD, ABPP, professor emeritus of Psychology,
Clinical Program BYU, adjunct associate professor of Psychiatry
School of Medicine, University of Utah SLC UT

"This workbook is accessible and helpful to both neophyte and advanced group therapy leaders. It takes a practical approach to integrating CBT and psychodrama in group. This offers a data-based methodology that also invites creativity through its experiential focus. The multiple case examples provide the clinician with clear idea of what it looks like in practice. A highly recommended read!"

Leann T. Diederich, PhD, Licensed Psychologist in Private Practice

"This innovative text integrates the theory and practice of Cognitive Behavioral Therapy (CBT) and Psychodrama, creating a new model – Cognitive Experiential Group Therapy (CEGT). CEGT brings together the best of both worlds – the evidence-based, systematic CBT approach offering multiple structured therapeutic instruments and psychodrama's experiential nature which emphasizes action, spontaneity, and creativity. The CEGT model offers a balanced approach of exploring emotions, thoughts, and behaviors through both experiential processes and participant's written self-reported data. Client examples with case conceptualizations are offered throughout the book depicting the CEGT model in action – furthermore, a dozen different worksheets are included, providing readers with practical resources for use in their work. A noteworthy strength of the revised edition is the addition of the CEGT model with adolescents and persons diagnosed with a social anxiety disorder. The authors have successfully integrated elements of theory, practice, and research making this a significant contribution to the literature. The incorporation of CBT with experiential theory and techniques enables action-oriented therapists to assimilate the wisdom from both CBT and psychodrama that is concretized in the CEGT model. This model is a valuable resource for enhancing the clinical practice of group therapy."

Scott Giacomucci, DSW, LCSW, director/founder at the
Phoenix Center for Experiential Trauma Therapy

Integrating CBT with Experiential Theory and Practice

A Group Therapy Workbook

Thomas W. Treadwell

With Deborah J. Dartnell,
Letitia E. Travaglini,
and Hanieh Abeditehrani

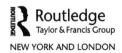

Routledge
Taylor & Francis Group

NEW YORK AND LONDON

First published 2021
by Routledge
52 Vanderbilt Avenue, New York, NY 10017

and by Routledge
2 Park Square, Milton Park, Abingdon, Oxon, OX14 4RN

Routledge is an imprint of the Taylor & Francis Group, an informa business

© 2021 Taylor & Francis

Library of Congress Cataloging-in-Publication Data
Names: Treadwell, Thomas W., author.
Title: Integrating CBT with experiential theory and practice : a
  group therapy workbook / Thomas W. Treadwell.
Description: New York, NY : Routledge, 2021. | Includes
  bibliographical references. |
Identifiers: LCCN 2020022401 (print) | LCCN 2020022402 (ebook) |
  ISBN 9780367856564 (hardback) | ISBN 9780367856557
  (paperback) | ISBN 9781003014379 (ebook)
Subjects: LCSH: Cognitive-experiential psychotherapy. |
  Drama—Therapeutic use. | Group psychotherapy.
Classification: LCC RC489.C63 T727 2021 (print) |
  LCC RC489.C63 (ebook) | DDC 616.89/152—dc23
LC record available at https://lccn.loc.gov/2020022401
LC ebook record available at https://lccn.loc.gov/2020022402

ISBN: 978-0-367-85656-4 (hbk)
ISBN: 978-0-367-85655-7 (pbk)
ISBN: 978-1-003-01437-9 (ebk)

Typeset in Sabon
by Apex CoVantage, LLC

Contents

About the Author

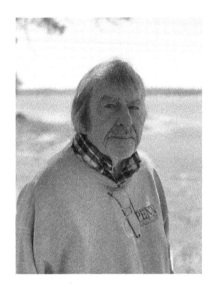

Thomas W. Treadwell, EdD, TEP, CGP, is a professor of psychology at West Chester University; clinical associate at the Center for Cognitive Therapy at the Perelman School of Medicine, University of Pennsylvania; editor for *The Group Psychologist*, Division 49, Society of Group Psychology and Group Psychotherapy, American Psychological Association; and a fellow of the American Society for Group Psychotherapy and Psychodrama. As a group therapist, he finds that effectiveness is better achieved when patients/clients and therapists work collaboratively as a therapeutic team. An interactive (cognitive and psychodramatic) action-oriented group focus is his treatment of choice in helping people readjust in modifying their communication and behavioral patterns to bring about healthy change. Cognitive group psychotherapy is a modality utilizing guided action and both psychodramatic and cognitive techniques to examine conflicts, predicaments, and crisis situations that are fathered/mothered in group or individual settings.

About the Contributors

Hanieh Abeditehrani, PhD, candidate in clinical psychology, is a member of the faculty of social and behavioral sciences at the University of Amsterdam in the Netherlands. Her PhD research is focused on comparing the effectiveness of psychodrama, cognitive behavioral group therapy, and the integration for social anxiety disorder in a randomized controlled trial. She does individual and group therapy in an intercultural mental health center in Amsterdam.

Deborah J. Dartnell, MSOD, MA, received her master's degree in organization development from American University and her master's in clinical psychology from West Chester University. She is an adjunct professor at West Chester University and has worked on cognitive experiential group therapy with Tom Treadwell for the past ten years. She has worked in community mental health as well as a hospital-based cancer center and is happiest when learning new skills and spending time with her grandchildren.

Letitia E. Travaglini, PhD, received her doctoral degree in Human Services Psychology, Clinical and Community/Applied Social Psychology from the University of Maryland, Baltimore (UMBC). She learned and studied CEGT while a student of Dr. Treadwell's at West Chester University. She currently is a clinician investigator for VA Capitol Health Care Network (VISN 5) Mental Illness Research, Education, and Clinical Center (MIRECC) (Baltimore, MD) and also a clinical health psychologist for the VA Maryland Health Care System (Baltimore, MD). Her clinical interests include individual and group therapy with adults with co-occurring mental and physical health disorders. Her research focus is on dissemination of evidence-based practices and the impact of social psychological factors impacting treatment engagement.

1 Introduction

The purpose of this workbook is to explain the techniques that are used and encountered by group members in the cognitive experiential group therapy (CEGT) model. This model incorporates cognitive behavioral and psychodramatic interventions to allow group members to identify and modify negative thinking, behavior, and interpersonal patterns. The workbook first provides a brief overview of cognitive behavioral therapy (CBT) and psychodrama, highlighting those concepts and techniques that are most relevant to CEGT session content. Next, it provides a description of CEGT and what group members should expect through their engagement in this therapy. An example of the CEGT session is then provided. The workbook then focuses on the use of CEGT with two special populations: adolescents and individuals with social anxiety disorder/social phobia. Several worksheets that are used by group members throughout CEGT are included in Appendix B.

CBT was established by Aaron T. Beck, MD (1967; Beck, Rush, Shaw, & Emery, 1979), and involves several techniques to challenge negative thought patterns and increase engagement in positive and success-based experiences. Psychodrama group therapy was created based on work by Jacob. L. Moreno, MD (1953), and involves experiential, interpersonal exercises to raise awareness and reduction of internal conflicts in order to change negative relational patterns. The CBT model is sometimes criticized for being overly structured and intellectually oriented (Woolfolk, 2000; Young & Klosko, 1994). As a result, some group therapists today use an approach based upon CBT or identify with a less structured approach called *eclectic* (Kellerman, 1992) that typically employs techniques that come from CBT and its related research. CBT is a robust, proven, and very effective treatment approach for many mental disorders, including the big ones like depression and anxiety (Association for Behavioral and Cognitive Therapies, 2008). Beck reports: "My employment of enactive, emotive strategies was influenced, no doubt, by psychodrama and Gestalt therapy" (Beck, 1991, p. 196). Psychodrama is an eclectic tool used to enhance cognitive and behavioral change. Several practitioners have worked to integrate CBT into the psychodramatic model by highlighting the ways CBT enhances psychodramatic exercises

(Boury, Treadwell, & Kumar, 2001; Treadwell & Kumar, 2002, 2005; Treadwell, Kumar, & Wright, 2004), adapting psychodrama to include the exploration of irrational beliefs (Kipper, 2002) and considering the way in which psychodrama could be considered a form of CBT (Baim, 2007; Shay, 2017; Treadwell, Travaglini, Reisch, & Kumar, 2011; Wilson, 2011). The blending of the two models yields a complementary approach to multiple problem-solving strategies (Treadwell et al., 2004):

- Both the CBT and psychodramatic models stress the discovery process through Socratic questioning. The use of certain structured CBT techniques (discussed within this manual) within the context of psychodrama provide ways to deepen self-reflection, problem-solving, and mood-regulation skills that can be rehearsed through psychodramatic exercises.
- Psychodramatic role-playing can provide individuals with opportunities to generate new ways of thinking and behaving. The spontaneity and creativity of individuals can be increased through the use of psychodramatic techniques, thus helping to produce alternative thoughts.

Prior to the group beginning, CEGT members go through a period of initial assessment. This assessment is done by completing a number of self-report forms and questionnaires, which are detailed within this workbook. This is necessary to establish the nature and severity of each group member's presenting concerns, possible presence of mental illness in past generations of one's family that may be impacting current functioning, and other relevant information (Leahy, 2003). Based on the collected information, the group director creates a common agenda for the group as well as personal agendas for each member of the group. Group members do not necessarily need to have the same presenting concern(s) or psychological disorder(s) to participate in the same CEGT group; it is more important that the severity of symptoms/disorders is similar (Leahy, 2003).

It is important to note that this workbook provides a very brief overview of concepts most relevant to CEGT session content. More detailed descriptions of CBT and psychodrama can be gathered from the following publications, as well as those in the References section of this workbook:

- Beck, J. S. (2011) *Cognitive Behavior Therapy: Basics and Beyond* (2nd ed.). New York: The Guilford Press.
- Beck, J. S. (2020) *Cognitive Behavioral Therapy: Basics and Beyond* (3rd ed.). New York: The Guilford Press.
- Karp, M., Holmes, P., & Tauvon, K. B. (1998). *The Handbook for Psychodrama*. New York: Routledge Press.
- Young, J. E., & Klasko, J. S. (1993). *Reinventing Your Life: The Breakthrough Program to End Negative Behavior and Feel Great Again*. New York: The Penguin Group.

2   Cognitive Behavioral Therapy

Cognitive behavioral therapy (CBT) is a therapeutic approach that is based on the cognitive behavioral model. This model focuses on a person's thoughts, feelings, and behaviors and takes a special interest in how they connect (Beck, 2011). CBT operates on the idea that what a person thinks affects how a person feels and how a person feels affects their behaviors. This is an ongoing cycle; often, the behaviors a person chooses will reinforce his or her thoughts and feelings. The following is an example:

Example A: Patty

- *Thought:* Patty has a belief that she is not pretty and therefore feels like no one would want to date her.
- *Feeling:* Patty feels sad, unloved, and lonely.
- *Behavior:* Patty chooses not to socialize because she is scared to be rejected and withdraws from people.
- *Ongoing cycle:* In turn, no one asks to date her because she does not allow herself to be put in social situations where she could meet potential partners. This reinforces her original thought that she is not pretty, but she does not realize that her behaviors are strengthening this thought and her feelings of sadness and loneliness.

Thoughts and Feelings

CBT encompasses a few general concepts about one's thought processes that comprise the core of the theory. These consist of schemas, core beliefs, cognitive distortions, intermediate beliefs, and automatic thoughts (Beck, 2011). All of these concepts impact an individual's thoughts (which, in turn, influence feelings and behaviors) and build upon each other to create dysfunctional thinking patterns (Figure 2.1). We will define each of these concepts next.

Schemas

Schemas describe a person's pattern of thoughts through underlying, pervasive organizational structures. Each person has a different way of

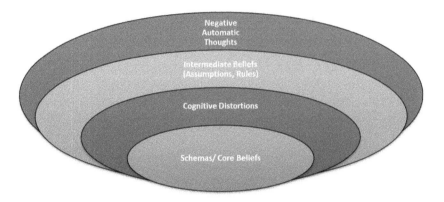

Figure 2.1 Thoughts and Beliefs Within the Cognitive Behavioral Model

organizing and understanding information as it is presented. This organizational scheme is essentially a framework for understanding the world. Schemas can be helpful to a person because they often serve as "shortcuts" to organizing the vast amounts of information each person is introduced to every day. These can also cause problems because people often leave out or ignore information that does not fit within their existing framework. Additionally, schemas tend to remain unchanged even when contradictory information is presented. This ignoring of contradictory or uncertain information can result in distorted information processing.

> **Example B:** A young boy named George may develop a schema for a dog. He knows that a four-legged, furry animal with a tail is called a dog. Now, when George encounters a horse for the first time, he will undoubtedly call this a dog. This is because he considers information that fits his present schema (e.g., four-legged, furry animal with a tail) and ignores contradictory information (e.g., mane and hooves).

An example like this may not create problems for George because this information may be corrected easily with new information given by an adult, therefore changing George's schema. However, when more rigid schemas are present, they can become increasingly problematic.

> **Example C:** Joe's parents were killed in an auto accident when he was 6 years old. His grandparents raised him until he was 15 years of age, when they became too ill to care for him. His aunt took over his care until he left for college. He married his high-school sweetheart; she left him after a few years for a close friend of theirs. Since then, he has had difficulty maintaining intimate,

long-term relationships and establishing new relationships. He reacts to minor signs of abandonment in an exaggerated way and feels excessive negative emotion. He might also remain in painful relationships despite the distress he may experience because he sees no other way to connect with others. He believes that, one way or another, everyone will leave him.

The main issue with schemas is that they are deeply rooted and often remain with a person as they grow older. For George, his schema is likely to change as he learns more about different animals. However, in situations like Joe's, these pervasive, negative beliefs may be harder to change and may lead to ongoing problems throughout life.

Young, Klosko, and Weishaar (2003) defines *schemas* as broad and persistent themes regarding oneself and one's relationship with others that are developed during childhood and elaborated throughout one's lifetime and are dysfunctional to a significant degree. Schemas, according to Young et al. (2003), develop in childhood as a result of negative experiences with parents, siblings, and peers. As a result of negative experiences, it is common to distort and view situations in our lives that support the validity of our schemas. Schemas remain dormant until they are activated by situations relevant to a specific schema. Young identified 18 schemas, categorized into five domains (see Table 2.1).

Core Beliefs

Core beliefs are the underlying feelings one has about himself or herself. There are three overarching negative core belief categories: "I'm helpless," "I'm worthless," and "I'm unlovable." Feeling this way about oneself colors the way a person thinks about himself or herself and others and causes a person to distort information to coincide with these beliefs. In her book *Cognitive Behavior Therapy: Basics and Beyond*, Dr. Judith Beck (2011) provides specific examples of helpless, worthless, and unlovable core beliefs, detailed in Table 2.2.

Let us go back to Example A about Patty, who thought she was not pretty and no one would date her. Based on this information, it is likely that she has an underlying core belief that she is *unlovable*. As a result, she bases her behaviors around this belief and will distort information to prove to herself that she is right (therefore strengthening this belief).

The following is an illustration of a *helpless* core belief: John failed his math test, activating negative thoughts of "I am inferior, a failure, a loser, not good enough, defective, and I don't measure up." The following is an example of a *worthless* core belief: Amy can't control her craving for painkillers and continues to use them regularly to cope with negative emotions and low self-esteem. Abusing pills activates negative thoughts of "I can't stand myself" and "I don't deserve to live." Thus,

Table 2.1 Young's Schemas

DOMAIN 1: DISCONNECTION AND REJECTION

The expectation that one's needs for security, safety, stability, nurturance, empathy, sharing of feelings, acceptance, and respect will not be met in a predictable manner. Typically, the person's family of origin is detached, cold, rejecting, withholding, lonely, explosive, unpredictable, or abusive.

1. **ABANDONMENT / INSTABILITY:** Perceived instability or unreliability of those available for bonding and support. Involves the sense that significant others will not be able to continue providing emotional support, connection, strength, or practical protection because they are emotionally unstable and unpredictable (e.g., angry outbursts), unreliable, or erratically present because they will die imminently or because they will abandon the person in favor of someone better.

2. **MISTRUST / ABUSE:** The expectation that others will hurt, abuse, humiliate, cheat, lie, manipulate, or take advantage. Usually involves the perception that the harm is intentional or the result of unjustified and extreme negligence. This may include the sense that one always ends up being cheated relative to others or "gets the short end of the stick."

3. **EMOTIONAL DEPRIVATION:** The expectation that one's desire for a normal degree of emotional support will not be adequately met by others. The three major forms of deprivation are:

   A. *Deprivation of nurturance:* Absence of attention, affection, warmth, or companionship.
   B. *Deprivation of empathy:* Absence of understanding, listening, self-disclosure, or mutual sharing of feelings from others.
   C. *Deprivation of protection:* Absence of strength, direction, or guidance from others.

4. **DEFECTIVENESS / SHAME:** The feeling that one is defective, bad, unwanted, inferior, or invalid in important respects or that one would be unlovable to significant others if exposed. May involve hypersensitivity to criticism, rejection, and blame; self-consciousness, comparisons, and insecurity around others; or a sense of shame regarding one's perceived flaws. These flaws may be private (e.g., selfishness, angry impulses, unacceptable sexual desires) or public (e.g., undesirable physical appearance, social awkwardness).

5. **SOCIAL ISOLATION / ALIENATION:** The feeling that one is isolated from the rest of the world, different from other people, and/or not part of any group or community.

DOMAIN 2: IMPAIRED AUTONOMY AND PERFORMANCE

Expectations about oneself and the environment that interfere with one's perceived ability to separate, survive, function independently, or perform successfully. Typically, the person's family of origin is enmeshed, undermining a child's confidence, overprotecting them, or failing to reinforce a child for performing competently outside the family.

6. **DEPENDENCE / INCOMPETENCE:** Belief that one is unable to handle everyday responsibilities in a competent manner without considerable help from others (e.g., take care of oneself, solve daily problems, exercise good judgment, tackle new tasks, make good decisions). Often presents as helplessness.

7. **VULNERABILITY TO HARM OR ILLNESS:** Exaggerated fear that imminent catastrophe will strike at any time and that one will be unable to prevent it. Fears focus on one or more of the following:

   A. *Medical catastrophes* (e.g., heart attacks, AIDS)
   B. *Emotional catastrophes* (e.g., going crazy)
   C. *External catastrophes* (e.g., elevator collapse, criminal victimization, plane crashes, earthquakes)

8. **ENMESHMENT / UNDEVELOPED SELF:** The excessive emotional involvement and closeness with one or more significant others (often parents) at the expense of full individuation or normal social development. Often involves the belief that at least one of the enmeshed individuals cannot survive or be happy without the constant support of the other. May also include feelings of being smothered by or fused with others, or insufficient individual identity. Often experienced as a feeling of emptiness and floundering, having no direction, or, in extreme cases, questioning one's existence.

9. **FAILURE:** The belief that one has failed, will inevitably fail, or is fundamentally inadequate relative to one's peers in areas of achievement (school, career, sports, etc.). Often involves beliefs that one is stupid, inept, untalented, ignorant, lower in status, or less successful than others.

DOMAIN 3: IMPAIRED LIMITS

A perceived deficiency in internal limits, responsibility to others, or long-term goal orientation. This can lead to difficulty respecting the rights of others, cooperating with others, making commitments, or setting and meeting realistic personal goals. Typically, family of origin is characterized by permissiveness, overindulgence, lack of direction, or a sense of superiority rather than appropriate confrontation, discipline, and limits in relation to taking responsibility, cooperating in a reciprocal manner, and setting goals. In some cases, the child may not have been pushed to tolerate normal levels of discomfort or may not have been given adequate supervision, direction, or guidance.

10. **ENTITLEMENT / GRANDIOSITY:** The belief that one is superior to other people, entitled to special rights and privileges, or not bound by the rules of reciprocity that guide normal social interaction. Often involves insistence that one should be able to do or have whatever one wants regardless of what is realistic, what others consider reasonable, or the cost to others; or an exaggerated focus on superiority (e.g., being among the most successful, famous, wealthy) in order to achieve power or control (not primarily for attention or approval). Sometimes includes excessive competitiveness toward, or domination of, others without empathy or concern for their needs or feelings: asserting one's power; forcing one's point of view; or controlling the behavior of others in line with one's own desires.

11. **INSUFFICIENT SELF-CONTROL / SELF-DISCIPLINE:** The pervasive difficulty or refusal to exercise sufficient self-control and frustration tolerance in order to achieve one's personal goals, or to restrain the excessive expression of one's emotions and impulses. In its milder form, one presents with an exaggerated emphasis on discomfort avoidance: avoiding pain, conflict, confrontation, responsibility, or overexertion at the expense of personal fulfillment, commitment, or integrity.

(Continued)

Table 2.1 (Continued)

DOMAIN 4: OTHER-DIRECTEDNESS

An excessive focus on the desires, feelings, and responses of others at the expense of one's own needs in order to gain love and approval, maintain one's sense of connection, or avoid retaliation. Usually involves suppression and lack of awareness regarding one's own anger and natural inclinations. Typically, family of origin is based on conditional acceptance: children must suppress important aspects of themselves in order to gain love, attention, and approval. In many such families, the parents' emotional needs and desires – or social acceptance and status – are valued more than the unique needs and feelings of each child.

12. **SUBJUGATION:** Excessive surrendering of control to others because one feels coerced, usually to avoid anger, retaliation, or abandonment. The two major forms of subjugation are:

   A. *Subjugation of needs:* Suppression of one's preferences, decisions, and desires.
   B. *Subjugation of emotions:* Suppression of emotional expression, especially anger. Usually involves the perception that one's own desires, opinions, and feelings are not valid or important to others. Frequently presents as excessive compliance, combined with hypersensitivity to feeling trapped. Generally, leads to a buildup of anger, manifested in maladaptive symptoms (e.g., passive-aggressive behavior, uncontrolled outbursts of temper, psychosomatic symptoms, withdrawal of affection, "acting out," and substance abuse).

13. **SELF-SACRIFICE:** Excessive focus on voluntarily meeting the needs of others in daily situations at the expense of one's own gratification. The most common reasons are to prevent causing pain to others, to avoid guilt from feeling selfish, and to maintain the connection with others perceived as needy. Often results from an acute sensitivity to the pain of others. Sometimes leads to a sense that one's own needs are not being adequately met and to resentment of those who are taken care of (overlaps with concept of codependency).

14. **APPROVAL-SEEKING / RECOGNITION-SEEKING:** Excessive emphasis on gaining approval, recognition, or attention from other people, or fitting in at the expense of developing a secure and true sense of self. One's sense of esteem is dependent primarily on the reactions of others rather than on one's own natural inclinations. Sometimes includes an overemphasis on status, appearance, social acceptance, money, or achievement as means of gaining approval, admiration, or attention (not primarily for power or control). Frequently results in major life decisions that are inauthentic or unsatisfying, or in hypersensitivity to rejection.

DOMAIN 5: OVERVIGILANCE AND INHIBITION

Excessive emphasis on suppressing one's spontaneous feelings, impulses, and choices, or on meeting rigid, internalized rules and expectations about performance and ethical behavior, often at the expense of happiness, self-expression, relaxation, close relationships, or health. Typically, family of origin is grim, demanding, and sometimes punitive, and performances, duty, perfectionism, following rules, hiding emotions, and avoiding mistakes predominate over pleasure, joy, and relaxation. There is usually an undercurrent of pessimism and worry, and a belief that things could fall apart if one fails to be vigilant and careful at all times.

15. **NEGATIVITY / PESSIMISM:** A pervasive, lifelong focus on the negative aspects of life (pain, death, loss, disappointment, conflict, guilt, resentment, unsolved problems, potential mistakes, betrayal, things that could go wrong, etc.) while minimizing or neglecting the positive or optimistic aspects. Usually includes an exaggerated expectation – in a wide range of work, financial, or interpersonal situations – that things will eventually go seriously wrong or that aspects of one's life that seem to be going well will ultimately fall apart. Usually involves an inordinate fear of making mistakes that might lead to financial collapse, loss, humiliation, or being trapped in a bad situation. Because potential negative outcomes are exaggerated, these individuals are frequently characterized by chronic worry, vigilance, complaining, or indecision.

16. **EMOTIONAL INHIBITION:** Excessive inhibition of spontaneous action, feeling, or communication, usually to avoid disapproval by others, feelings of shame, or losing control of one's impulses. The most common areas of inhibition involve:

    A. *Inhibition of anger and aggression*
    B. *Inhibition of positive impulses (e.g., joy, affection, sexual excitement, play)*
    C. *Difficulty expressing vulnerability or communicating freely about feelings, needs, etc.*
    D. *Excessive emphasis on rationality while disregarding emotions*

17. **UNRELENTING STANDARDS / HYPERCRITICALNESS:** The underlying belief that one must strive to meet very high internalized standards of behavior and performance, usually to avoid criticism. Typically results in feelings of pressure or difficulty slowing down and being hypercritical toward oneself and others. One must exhibit significant impairment in pleasure, relaxation, health, self-esteem, sense of accomplishment, or satisfying relationships. Unrelenting standards typically present as:

    A. *Perfectionism, including inordinate attention to detail or an underestimate of how good one's own performance is relative to the norm*
    B. *Rigid rules and "shoulds" in many areas of life, including unrealistically high moral, ethical, cultural, or religious precepts*
    C. *Preoccupation with time and efficiency so that more can be accomplished*

18. **PUNITIVENESS:** The belief that people should be harshly punished for making mistakes. This involves the tendency to be angry, intolerant, punitive, and impatient with those people (including oneself) who do not meet one's expectations or standards. Usually includes difficulty forgiving mistakes in oneself or others because of a reluctance to consider extenuating circumstances, allow for human imperfection, or empathize with feelings.

Adapted from Young, J. E., Klosko, J. S., & Weishaar, M. E. (2003). *Schema therapy: A practitioner's guide.* New York: The Guilford Press.

Table 2.2 Examples of Core Beliefs

Helpless	Unlovable	Worthless
"I am powerless."	"I am unlikable."	"I am worthless."
"I am out of control."	"I am undesirable."	"I am unacceptable."
"I am weak."	"I am uncared for."	"I am bad, crazy, broken,
"I am needy."	"I am unworthy."	nothing, a waste."
"I am inadequate."	"I am defective."	"I am hurtful, dangerous,
"I am a failure."	"I am bound to be	toxic, and evil."
"I am not good enough."	rejected."	"I don't deserve to live."
	"I am different."	

pervasive negative beliefs are deeply held core ideas that influence thinking patterns, interpretations of events, and behavioral responses. When activated, these ideas trigger unhelpful response mechanisms and mood or anxiety symptoms.

The next section of this workbook will describe two aspects of a person's thought processes that are influenced by underlying schemas and core beliefs: cognitive distortions and automatic thoughts.

Cognitive Distortions

People will often distort information to fit their core beliefs and schemas; this is known as a *cognitive distortion*. Twelve categories of "cognitive distortions" have been identified and defined based on a person's tendency to change or ignore information with which they are provided (Beck, 2011). While people can distort information to become more positive, cognitive distortions in CBT are negative in nature; that is, people will see people, places, or objects as unhealthy or negative. There are many types of cognitive distortions (see Appendix A for a complete list). A few of the most common ones are black-and-white thinking, overgeneralization, catastrophizing, and personalization. We will review these four cognitive distortions in more detail next.

Black-and-white thinking (often referred to as all-or-nothing thinking) occurs when a person only sees one extreme of a spectrum. For example:

- If a man is not perfect in one thing, he will think he is a failure at all things; he believes he is either a success or a failure and there can be nothing in between.
- If a high-achieving student gets a B on a test, this must mean that she is a failure because she did not get an A.

Overgeneralization occurs when a person takes one (bad) situation and sees it as a never-ending pattern of defeat. For example:

- If a teenage boy gets turned down for a date by one girl, he may think, "No one ever wants to date me." It may be that this is the first girl he has ever asked out, but he will take this instance and apply it with a large paintbrush.

Catastrophizing occurs when a person exaggerates the significance of an event. People who catastrophize tend to view situations worse than they actually are. For example:

- A couple has a simple disagreement, and one person views it as the end of their relationship.
- An employee makes a minor mistake and thinks he will be fired.

Personalization occurs when people feel that everything that happens to them is aimed directly at them when it may have nothing to do with them. Personalization can be seen as a selfish viewpoint where people see themselves as the center of events around them. For example:

- When the person in front of the businessman does not hold the door, it would be "because people are always mean to me."
- If this man is late for a meeting, he may take complete blame for the meeting not going as planned even though this was not his fault.

Automatic Thoughts

When any situation arises, people tend to have thoughts that pop into their heads without warning. In CBT, these thoughts are referred to as *automatic thoughts*. They are the quick, initial thoughts that go through a person's mind when a negative event happens, often related to the gut-level reaction one has toward the event.

> **Example D:** Susan wakes up and realizes that her alarm clock did not sound. Automatically, she has thoughts such as "I might get fired!" or "What excuse can I give my boss this time?" or "I am going to be late for my conference call."

These thoughts tend to fit within the person's existing schemas and core beliefs. If Susan has a schema that she is not competent and a core belief that she is helpless, then she will more than likely incorporate a cognitive distortion, such as catastrophizing, into her automatic thoughts. These thoughts are also coupled with the feelings she experiences as a result of waking up late for work.

Challenge Thinking Through Thought Records

Automatic Thought Records (ATRs) (Greenberger & Padesky, 1995, 2015) are useful CBT-based tools for challenging and correcting automatic thoughts and core beliefs. ATRs call on an individual to recognize the thoughts and feelings around a negative situation and begin challenging the underlying, intermediate beliefs fueling these thoughts and emotions. Let's use Susan's example as a way to break down the components of an ATR:

Situation	Moods (mood rating out of 10)	Automatic thoughts
Wakes up late for work because the alarm clock did not sound.	Anxious (9) Worried (8) Upset (7) Frantic (10)	I might get fired. What excuse can I give my boss this time? I am going to be late for my conference call. **I cannot do anything right.**

At times, it is helpful to rate how strongly an emotion is felt. As seen in the table, Susan was able to rate her emotions on a 1–10 scale (10 being the most extreme) of how intense her emotions were at the time of the situation. Following the mood ratings, she was able to identify the automatic thoughts she had about being late for work. The last sentence, "I cannot do anything right," really highlights how Susan feels about herself. Often, when we take the time to pay attention to our automatic thoughts, we realize how we feel about ourselves. This thought – "I cannot do anything right" – would be termed her *hot thought*. The hot thought typically reflects the intermediate, core belief that is explaining her automatic thoughts and feelings in this situation; specifically, Susan probably has a core belief that falls into the *helpless* category.

At this point, Susan may begin feeling upset about this belief. Stopping at this point could strengthen her core belief of helplessness. In CBT, the goal is to begin challenging these automatic thoughts and intermediate beliefs so that people are able to create more positive beliefs about themselves and their experiences. What is typically done, then, is to begin generating concrete examples that both support and go against this intermediate belief that she cannot do anything right. These examples may be pulled from any time throughout the person's life. First, she will review any evidence that supports her hot thought. Then, she will review the evidence against the hot thought as a way to begin challenging her core belief:

Automatic thoughts	Evidence that supports the hot thought	Evidence that does not support the hot thought
I might get fired. What excuse can I give my boss this time? I am going to be late for my conference call. **I cannot do anything right.**	1. I am late for work for the second time this month. 2. I got a verbal warning about being on time. 3. I didn't do well in college. 4. Time management has always been a problem. 5. I was late to take a major test and failed. 6. My family hounds me for regularly being late to events.	1. Although I was late two times, I was on time 29 times. 2. I graduated college. 3. I raised two children alone. 4. I was never late to my other job. 5. I always complete my work. 6. I am often the first person called upon for important tasks at work. 7. I have never been fired from a job.

While focusing on the evidence for and against is helpful at starting to break down the intermediate belief ("I cannot do anything right") and weaken the core belief (helplessness), we do not want to just stop here. Next, we want to create a *balanced thought* using the evidence for and against the hot thought. A balanced thought is one that combines the core belief with a more positive view of the person and/or the situation to create a healthier, more balanced way of thinking. For Susan, her balanced thought must recognize that she does some things wrong, but that it does not mean she "cannot do anything right." Once a balanced thought is created and rated, the person then re-rates the moods initially experienced to see if this process has reduced or increased the strength of these feelings. In Susan's example, she would again rate her feelings of anxious, worried, upset, and frantic.

Balanced thought	Mood
Although I was late today, I am accountable and I take care of my professional responsibilities. (7)	Anxious (6) Worried (6) Upset (3) Frantic (7)

As you can see, this process of talking oneself through a tough situation often leads to decreased negative feelings by changing the way the person thinks. It is also helpful to rate how much you believe your balanced thought on a scale of 1 (lowest) to 10 (highest).

ATRs will be used often during cognitive psychodrama group therapy. They allow an individual to assess a situation and make a balanced

Table 2.3 Example Automatic Thought Record

Situation	Moods	Automatic Thoughts (Images)	Evidence That Supports The Hot Thought	Evidence That Does Not Support The Hot Thought	Alternative/ Balanced Thoughts	Rate Moods Now
My best friend moved back to New York over the weekend.	Sad (10) Upset (10) Helpless (8) Lonely (9)	Everyone leaves me! People don't want to be around me! You were my best friend, and you are leaving me. I am not lovable! I don't matter to people! I am invisible! I'm a piece of shit. I'm worthless. **I am bound to be alone (abandonment).**	1. I lost a lot of friendships in college because of people moving. 2. I didn't talk to my dad for almost eight months because of my ex-boyfriend. 3. I'm not home as much as I should be, and when I am home, I am holed up in my room doing homework. 4. My little sister didn't know who I was until she was 2 or 3. 5. I have no friends in the area. 6. My parents divorced, and I was to blame. 7. I had a strained relationship with my dad. 8. My mother doesn't really know who I am. 9. I was always left out in my family.	1. I have one absolutely amazing friend, who lives in Florida, that I have been in contact with for eight years. 2. My little sister looks up to me now. 3. My dad is always there for me. 4. I am about to graduate from college. 5. I have a potential job when I graduate. 6. I have more than one professor writing me a letter of recommendation. 7. My friend (the one who moved) keeps telling me he isn't more than a phone call away.	Even though he moved, my friend is there for me. (7) Even though people are in and out of my life, the ones that matter are here. (9) Even though I feel alone sometimes, I have a good relationship with my dad, my little sister, and my best friend. (6)	Sad (8) Upset (8) Helpless (7) Lonely (8)

Adapted from Greenberger, D., & Padesky, C. (1995, 2015). *Mind over mood: Change how you feel by changing the way you think.* New York, NY: The Guilford Press.

Table 2.4 Example Dysfunctional Thought Record

Date and time	Situation	Automatic thought(s)	Emotion(s)	Adaptive response	Outcome
	1. Actual event, stream of thoughts, or daydreams or recollection that led to the unpleasant emotion. 2. What (if any) distressing physical sensations did you have?	1. What thought(s) and/or image(s) went through your mind? 2. How much did you believe each one at the time?	1. What emotion(s) (sad/anxious/angry/etc.) did you feel at the time? 2. How intense (0–100%) was the emotion?	1. (Optional) What cognitive distortions did you make? 2. Use questions at bottom to compose a response to the automatic thought(s). 3. How much do you believe each response?	1. How much do you believe each automatic thought? 2. What emotion(s) do you feel now? How intense (0–100%) is the emotion? 3. What will you do (or did you do)?
July 1, 2019, 8 a.m.	Woke up late because my alarm clock didn't go off. Felt sick to my stomach.	I won't make it to work on time! What will my boss think? How do I explain this? I look irresponsible. Maybe I am irresponsible. I don't deserve this job. Maybe I am not competent for this position.	Nervous: 90% Anxious: 95% Upset: 80% Rushed: 100%	A. Cognitive distortions: 　1. Overgeneralization 　2. Black-and-white thinking 　3. Catastrophizing B. Responses: 　1. This is a one-time event. I did not have control of this. 　2. Worst that can happen is I get yelled at. Best is that no one cares. Most realistic is that my boss would be upset but move on. 　3. The effect of me believing this automatic thought is that I blow everything out of proportion and believe this one mistake makes me incompetent. 　4. I should begin to look at events as isolated incidents and not get overwhelmed. C. Believe each response: 90%	1. Believe my automatic thoughts: 50% 2. Emotions 　Nervous: 40% 　Anxious: 50% 　Upset: 50% 　Rushed: 80% 3. Called my boss and calmly explained the situation.

Questions to help compose an adaptive response: (1) What is the evidence that the automatic thought is true? Not true? (2) Is there an alternative explanation? (3) What's the worst that could happen? How could I cope? What's the best that could happen? What's the most realistic outcome? (4) What's the effect of my believing the automatic thought? What could be the effect of my changing my thinking? (5) What should I do about it? (6) If _____ [friend's name] was in the situation and had this thought, what would I tell him or her?

Thought Record. Adapted from Cognitive behavior therapy worksheet packet. © 2011 by Judith Beck. Bala Cynwyd, PA: Beck Institute for Cognitive Behavior Therapy.

decision about the event. The ATR is a step-by-step process that allows a person to really think through the thoughts and feelings associated with a given situation. In time, it will not be necessary to write down the information, as the process will become second nature.

Another way to talk yourself down from a stressful situation is by using a technique called a Dysfunctional Thought Record (DTR) (Beck et al., 1979). The DTR is a self-reflection strategy that aids in improving problem-solving skills and mood regulation. As a reminder, our emotional state is directly tied to the way we think. By changing the way you think about an event or a challenge, you put yourself in a better position to change the feelings you experience. Emotional distress is caused by disordered thinking. These thinking errors, in turn, are caused by habits of thinking that are exaggerated. The DTR helps you identify these errors so that you can replace them with thoughts that accurately reflect reality. DTRs are typically used more as a solution-based technique, allowing a person to integrate various cognitive techniques learned in therapy. For example, when a person notices they are having strong negative emotions, they may ask themselves: "When that happened, what just went through my mind? What cognitive distortion am I experiencing?"

Behavioral Interventions

Behavioral interventions are used in CBT to combat the lack or avoidance of physical and/or pleasurable activity that we often experience as a result of low mood, anxiety, and other psychological distress. It can help increase a person's social life, decrease avoidance, and challenge negative thoughts. These activities are designed to build confidence in one's abilities and improve self-esteem while decreasing depression, anxiety, and feelings of helplessness and unlovability.

Behavioral interventions are regularly used in the therapeutic process. Table 2.5 includes examples of behavioral interventions and a brief description of each. These are activities you may be asked to engage in during your time in cognitive psychodrama group therapy, so it will be helpful to familiarize yourself with them.

Summary/Review

- Cognitive behavioral therapy (CBT) is a type of treatment that focuses on the way a person thinks, feels, and behaves.
- The "cognitive" component of CBT is comprised of schemas, core beliefs, cognitive distortions, and automatic thoughts:
  - Schemas are a person's pattern of thought and are ways to organize information.
  - Core beliefs are ways in which a person feels about himself or herself. The negative core beliefs fall into three categories: helpless, unlovable, and worthless.

Table 2.5 Example Behavioral Interventions

Intervention	Examples
Activity Monitoring and Scheduling	• Monitor daily activities and rate the degree of pleasure and accomplishment for each activity on a scale of 1 (lowest) to 10 (highest). As a person becomes aware of how much time they spend on low-pleasure or low-accomplishment activities, the therapist and group members will help him or her gradually replace these with higher pleasure and accomplishment activities. • Over time, it will be important to start scheduling into the week the behavioral treatment goals identified at the beginning of therapy. • It may be necessary to anticipate obstacles to achieving the goals, to challenge those obstacles, and to develop strategies to respond to unforeseen events. • See Appendix B for a blank activity schedule.
Graded Activity Exposure – Stepladder Approach Fear Hierarchy	• When scheduling activities, improve success rates by breaking down large, unrealistic goals into smaller, more manageable pieces. It is often important to consider realistically what you can accomplish now. • See Appendix B for blank goal-setting and graded exposure worksheets. • Anxious people avoid feared situations because they often have catastrophic beliefs that experiencing those situations will harm them. For example, a man with panic disorder may avoid exercise because he perceives light-headedness and rapid heart rate as signs of imminent heart attack. Avoiding exercise to prevent the feared symptoms perpetuates his catastrophic beliefs. • It is often helpful to expose yourself to feared situations or objects for small amounts of time. An alternative would be to create a fear hierarchy (make a list of fearful situations/objects and order the list from least to most anxiety provoking), then begin working your way through each item on the list. • See Appendix B for a blank fear hierarchy worksheet.
In Vivo Exposure	• Confront the avoided object or situation. For example, the therapist may show a woman with needle phobia pictures of needles, followed by actual needles themselves, and then she may be asked to touch a needle, hold a needle, etc., until her anxiety gradually diminishes.
Imaginal Exposure	• This involves asking a person to imagine himself or herself in a feared situation and to manipulate the images to build a sense of mastery. If he or she stops the image at the moment of highest arousal, he or she is instructed to "continue to play the film forward" by asking, "What happens next?" This approach shows the person that he or she can cope with difficult situations.

- Cognitive distortions are exaggerated and irrational thoughts. Some of the more common cognitive distortions are black-and-white thinking, overgeneralization, catastrophizing, and personalization.
- Automatic thoughts are reflexive thoughts that pop into a person's mind when a situation occurs.
- Automatic Thought Records (ATRs) allow you to assess a situation and make a balanced decision about the event.
- Dysfunctional Thought Records (DTRs) are a way to self-reflect and improve problem-solving skills after a stressful situation.

- Behavioral interventions are used to increase social skills and decrease avoidance. They challenge negative thoughts and help provide mastery over difficult situations.
- In cognitive experiential group therapy (CEGT), you may be asked to complete ATRs and participate in behavioral interventions.

3 Psychodrama Therapy

Psychodrama is a method that integrates the modes of CBT with dimensions of experiential and participatory involvement. Psychodrama sessions are individually focused but utilize other members of the group to help act out situations in the person's life. According to Blatner (1996), psychodrama emphasizes the "doing" of an interaction or situation (as opposed to only talking about/through it) in a way that engages the physical body and imagination as if the situation was happening in the present moment. This procedure or technique brings into consciousness many ideas and feelings not generally assessed through simply talking through the situation. The psychodramatic protocol has three components: the "warming up phase" (preparing the protagonist), the "action phase" (locating the conflicting situation and acting it out), and the "sharing phase" (involving group members to contribute their personal responses to the protagonist).

Psychodramatic Roles and Techniques

There are some common terms used for psychodrama participants. A partial list of frequently utilized psychodramatic roles and techniques is included in this chapter to assist in learning about the role(s) of each person. A common technique is role reversal, which includes either exploring conflicting roles within ourselves or assuming roles of others. Role reversal requires one to assume the "other" role and to feel and imagine how it affects one's perspective. Thus, role reversal allows an individual to gain insight and develop the capacity for empathy with self and others (Kellerman, 1994). By closely recreating real-life situations and acting them out in the present, clients have the opportunity to evaluate their behavior and more deeply understand a particular situation in their lives and the lives of others. See Table 3.1 for a list of common roles and techniques used in psychodrama.

Traditional psychodrama is conceptualized in terms of three main techniques: warming up, action, and sharing. There is no dearth

Table 3.1 Common Psychodramatic Roles and Techniques

Role	Description
Protagonist	This is the term for the "main character," or the role of the person who is pursuing a problem to gain insight in order to develop an alternative response in his or her life.
Double	The double joins the protagonist in his or her portrayal of himself or herself. This second actor assumes the role of an "auxiliary ego" (see next), which reveals hidden parts of the protagonist's behavior, by acting as him or her. The double expresses the thoughts and feelings the protagonist is repressing or not expressing.
Auxiliary Ego(s)	A group member is selected to play the role of another person in the situation that may be a partial cause for some of the protagonist's distress or concerns. In addition, the auxiliary ego will serve the purpose of identifying thoughts and feelings that the protagonist may be experiencing but not outwardly expressing. More than one auxiliary ego may be chosen to bring forward to express different thoughts or behaviors.
Cognitive Double	The cognitive double expresses the positive thoughts the protagonist is thinking, feeling, or repressing to the group. This technique explores and exposes the irrational beliefs and distorted thoughts/thinking of the protagonist.
De-roling	When enactments are concluded, the protagonist and other actors (auxiliaries) disengage from the roles that were played.

Technique	Description
Mirroring	The protagonist is asked to act out an experience. After this, the protagonist steps out of the scene and watches as another actor (auxiliary) steps into the role and recreates the scene. Afterward, the protagonist is asked to comment on the action and/or reenter the scene.
Soliloquy	The protagonist speaks his or her thoughts aloud (inner stream of consciousness is verbally expressed) in order to build self-knowledge and self-confidence.
Role Reversal	The protagonist is asked to portray another person (reverse roles) or play another part of himself or herself while an auxiliary ego portrays the protagonist in the particular scene. The protagonist and auxiliary will frequently switch roles and take on each other's roles several times during a session. This not only prompts the protagonist to think as the other person but also has some of the benefits of mirroring, as the client sees himself or herself portrayed by the second actor (auxiliary).
Role-Training	The protagonist practices a role, simulates a situation, and tries different answers, alternatives, or behaviors to a role that was not making a difference. The aim is to create situations for the development and training of certain role(s) in conditions very close to the real situation yet in a protected way.

Technique	Description
Role-Taking	The protagonist assumes a role, one that is not part of his or her ordinary life, and is placed in action with a narrow or broad description of how the role is portrayed.
Interview in Role Reversal	Prior to the role-play, the protagonist will often be interviewed as themselves and as the other individuals (antagonists) in the situation. Taking on the role of others allows second actors the opportunity to get a better understanding of the antagonist in the situation.
Empty Chair	Rather than having an auxiliary take on the confused role of the protagonist, an empty chair represents that position.
Sharing	Immediately following an enactment, group members share with the protagonist (and others) in what ways the drama reminded them of aspects in their own lives. Auxiliaries share how they felt playing the role as well as how they felt after they were de-roled.
Future Projection	Identifying a specific scene of an upcoming situation in the future. The event is explored in action (e.g., a job interview, apprehension about resigning from a current position).

Note: For a detailed list of psychodramatic roles and techniques, see Moreno (1953) and Blatner (2000).

of techniques that may be applied in the three phases (see Kumar & Treadwell, 1986). The versatility of psychodrama stems from the variety of techniques that have been borrowed or adapted from various individual and group psychotherapy modalities. With the increasing popularity of CBT techniques, especially those developed by Beck and his colleagues (see Beck et al., 1979; Beck, 1995) in the treatment of anxiety and depression in individual psychotherapy, there is an increasing interest in applying techniques unique to the cognitive behavioral model to group modalities, including psychodrama. Practitioners of traditional psychodrama are beginning to borrow or adapt techniques from CBT.

Psychodrama is a systematized method of role-playing enabling an individual, within a group setting, to explore the psychosocial dimensions of conflicts, problems, interpersonal relationships, and life situations through *enactment* rather than solely verbal means. This is accomplished utilizing both verbal and somatic (body awareness) methods (Fong, 2007). Psychodrama is, in one way, unique from other therapies; although it utilizes verbal communication, it is not overly dependent on verbal modes of treatment. By physically reenacting experiences, the past is brought into the here and now, permitting one to process memories with the therapist's/director's guidance along with the participation of group members with similar traumas (Kipper, 1998).

The CBT techniques utilized in a group therapy setting are sufficiently flexible for application during any of the three phases of psychodrama. The technique deepens traditional psychodrama not only by emphasizing the cathartic aspects of psychotherapy but also by incorporating the more goal-focused, problem-solving aspects of CBT.

Both the CBT and psychodramatic models stress the discovery process through Socratic questioning. For example, the use of certain structured, goal-oriented CBT techniques – for example, the Automatic Thought Record (ATR) and the downward arrow technique – within the context of a psychodrama session provides additional ways of stimulating the development of self-reflection, problem-solving, and mood-regulation skills. The blending of the two models yields a complementary eclectic approach to multiple problem-solving strategies.

Moreno (1972) describes psychodrama as the "scientific exploration of truth through dramatic method" (p. 12). Beck (1991) reports: "My employment of enactive, emotive strategies was influenced, no doubt, by psychodrama and Gestalt therapy" (p. 196). The psychodramatic approach, according to Blatner (2000), is a method for exploring psychological and social problems by having group members enact relevant events in their lives instead of talking about them. This process is grounded in principles of creativity, spontaneity, group dynamics, and role theory in order to evoke cognitive, emotional, and behavioral responses. The notion is that a new perspective will be achieved through the client understanding their roles in life and the ways they interact with others, coupled with obstacles that create challenges in their lives. Both Moreno and Beck had ideas that were initially seen as rebellious or novel compared with mainstream thought at the time. Psychodrama is an eclectic tool to enhance cognitive and behavioral change.

A core tenet of psychodrama, according to Schact (2007), is Moreno's theory of "spontaneity-creativity." Moreno posits that spontaneity is a physical, mental, and interpersonal process given direction by creativity. According to Moreno, creativity is a form of action, the act of creation, whereas spontaneity is the readiness to create (Sarol-Kulka, 2004). Moreno said: "Spontaneity operates in the present, here and now: it induces the individual to respond adequately to a novel situation, allowing an individual to respond creatively to a conflicting situation with a new and different response to an old negative situation" (as cited in Sarol-Kulka, 2004); in other words, an individual responds creatively to a conflicting situation (Blatner & Cukier, 2007). By encouraging an individual to address a problem in a creative way, reacting spontaneously and based on aspiration, they may begin to discover new solutions to problems in their lives and learn new roles.

Assimilating psychodramatic and cognitive behavioral theory and techniques in a group therapy setting cultivates the following objectives:

- Reduction of stress, anxiety, and tension.
- Minimization of distorted cognitive perceptions.
- Manifestation of unconscious motivation (hidden or unknown desires).
- Strengthening of self-esteem.
- Increased socialization and social adaptability skills.
- Increased awareness of self-understanding coupled with an acquisition of new insights about self.
- Interrupting the cyclical, repetitive, and maladaptive reactions to negative situations.
- Implementing positive adaptive behavioral patterns to negative scenarios.
- Understanding resilience and one's ability to overcome adverse events.
- Initiating positive interpersonal relationships

Briefly, the cognitive behavioral group psychodramatic modality emphasizes constructivist theory, holding both a person's individual sense of reality and the meaning found in life to be constructed from life experience. As a result of the model's experiential nature, much of its power lies in the simultaneous involvement of three major human modes: negative thinking (cognitive), action (behavior), and affect (emotions). The model provides immediate and objective feedback to group members, giving them flexible and adaptable tools. One of the most important elements of integrating CBT and psychodrama is that they are data based. From a constructivist perspective, group members keep track of their dysfunctional thoughts, depression scores, anxiety scores, and helplessness scores from session to session. They are able to see changes resulting from group therapy, making the therapeutic process a tractable one. The combination of CBT and psychodramatic techniques helps provide a balance between an exploration of emotionally laden situations and a more concrete, data-based problem-solving process.

Summary/Review

- Psychodrama is a method that integrates the modes of CBT with dimensions of experiential and participatory involvement.
- The psychodramatic protocol has three components: the "warming up phase" (preparing the protagonist), the "action phase" (locating the conflicting situation and acting it out), and the "sharing phase" (involving group members to contribute their personal responses to the protagonist).
- Psychodrama is a systematized method of role-playing enabling an individual, within a group setting, to explore the psychosocial dimensions of conflicts, problems, interpersonal relationships, and life situations through *enactment* rather than solely verbal means.
- Both the CBT and psychodramatic models stress the discovery process through Socratic questioning.

- A core tenet of psychodrama is Moreno's theory of "spontaneity-creativity."
- The cognitive behavioral group psychodramatic modality emphasizes constructivist theory, holding both a person's individual sense of reality and the meaning found in life to be constructed from life experiences.

4 Cognitive Experiential Group Therapy

Cognitive experiential group therapy (CEGT) combines both CBT and psychodramatic techniques to resolve distress and promote change. In applying the various CBT and psychodramatic techniques within the group model, it is important that all members understand CEGT and feel comfortable implementing techniques in group. CBT and action techniques can be used effectively within the context of psychodrama. In our experience, teenagers, adults, college students, and clinical populations respond well to this approach and, as a result, are able to develop an awareness of their dysfunctional thought patterns and beliefs that play an important role in mood regulation. CEGT adds a new dimension to both the fields of cognitive behavior and group therapy and is built on a proven efficacious model. The integration of these methods may be beneficial for clients who have not responded to more traditional approaches.

The group format is, foremost, a problem-solving approach for working through various interpersonal, occupational, educational, psychological, and health-related conflicts. The CEGT environment provides a supportive and safe climate to practice new thinking and behaviors (Treadwell et al., 2004). As such, time is spent in the first one to two sessions creating a safe and secure environment for the group where group members can freely share their concerns. The techniques employed in CEGT go above and beyond typical group therapy sessions. Table 4.1 identifies the differences between cognitive psychodrama group therapy and traditional group (talk) therapy.

Session Format

Each group session in CEGT is divided into three sections that are typical in psychodramatic interventions: *warm-up*, *action*, and *sharing*. The first portion (warm-up) of CEGT utilizes many CBT techniques. It focuses on identifying upsetting situations, automatic negative thoughts, and triggered moods; writing balanced thoughts to counter negative automatic thoughts; and recognizing distortions in thinking and imprecise interpretations of difficult situations. The second portion (action) employs

Table 4.1 CEGT Versus Traditional Group Therapy

Cognitive Experiential Group Therapy	Traditional Group (Talk) Therapy
Systematic method of collaborative group therapy. Deep action method challenging dysfunctional belief system.	**Generalized** approach to assist others in groups. More superficial and generalized. Can focus on specific disorders.
Oriented toward in-depth personal exploration, catharsis, insight, problem-solving, and behavior change. Encourages expression of deep feelings and beliefs.	Not oriented toward deep catharsis or expression of deep emotions. Not a problem-solving method.
Oriented toward revisiting the past, freeing persons from effects of previous traumatic situations (usually the origin of many maladaptive schemas), and adjusting to the present/future.	Oriented toward future situations and rehearsal of specific behavioral responses or approaches to anticipated situations. Ordinarily not directed toward the past.
Oriented toward personality, relationships, and maladaptive beliefs.	Oriented toward specific behavioral problems. Concentrates on social skills, behavioral modification, and training for social interaction (social phobia).
Deals with the effect of past on present behavior. Deals with conflicts within one's self as well as interpersonal conflicts. One's belief system is challenged and reorganized.	Usually concentrates on interpersonal interactive situations and is not intrapsychic.
Deals directly with personal life history and private problems (secret beliefs).	Usually focuses on aspects of the individual's social roles.
Very direct and collaborative method. Is self-disclosing and has built-in ways of dealing with exposure.	More indirect. May be less exposing.
Tests reactions/behavior to new situations within group setting. Utilizes behavioral experiments.	Usually does not test during life of group.

psychodramatic techniques such as role-playing, role reversal, and mir-roring, which facilitate the process of examining various conflicting situ-ations individuals experience within the context of a group. This enables group members to better understand the nature of negative thoughts trig-gered by situations and their effects on moods. The last stage (sharing) is for auxiliaries and group members to share their experiences with the protagonist. Next, we go into more details about the three phases of CEGT sessions.

Warm-up

During the warm-up phase, a protagonist is identified; typically, a group member will volunteer. We first utilize the Automatic Thought Record (ATR) to identify automatic thoughts, core beliefs, and schemas. The situation used for the action phase is often selected based on what was discussed in the ATR, either the specific situation used in the ATR or another, similar situation. It is preferred that the chosen situation is one that is unresolved or recurring so that the protagonist can apply what was learned in session to real-world resolution. Next, a genogram will be completed in order to pull out further information regarding the protagonist's past as it relates to his or her family of origin. To further enhance the picture of the protagonist's support system, a social atom may also be developed. Information on how to complete a genogram and develop the social atom will be explained later in this workbook. The warm-up also includes setting up the psychodrama. Additional people who are involved in the situation are identified, interviews are conducted in role reversal, and group members are chosen to take on additional roles in the situation (auxiliaries and doubles). This sets the stage for action, during which a protagonist is encouraged to enter into a state of mind where they can be present in their situation and aware of the current moment.

Action

During the action section of the psychodrama session, the enactment of a situation takes place. It is during the actual psychodrama that tech-niques such as mirroring, soliloquy, and role reversal occur. It is possible that the situation or focus of the psychodrama will change as the action phase progresses; for example, what begins as a role-play of a conflict between friends may switch to focusing on internal conflict within the protagonist. Psychodrama is helpful in pulling out additional conflicts and core beliefs that may not have been initially revealed through the ATR. The action phase continues until it is determined that there is reso-lution: either the identified problem is resolved, or the internal conflict within the protagonist is reduced.

Sharing

Finally, in the sharing phase, the various auxiliaries and other group members share their empathy and experiences with the protagonist of the scene. Doubles and auxiliaries describe what it felt like in those roles and in the role of the protagonist (if role reversal was used). Giving advice to the protagonist is detrimental; only sharing experiences and empathy is necessary. An additional component of this stage, processing, follows the sharing portion in order to examine the techniques utilized during the session. This is followed by discussion from the protagonist, auxiliaries, and audience. During processing, group members comment on the action and investigate why certain techniques were applied.

At this stage, the director may provide additional guidance to the protagonist regarding ways to begin resolving the actual situation in real life. It is usually the case that the protagonist will be asked to complete a homework assignment that will then be reviewed at the next session. See Appendix B for a blank homework worksheet.

Use of Assessment and Thought Record Data

One of the most important elements of CEGT is that it is data based. Group members record their dysfunctional thoughts; keep track of their depression, anxiety, and hopelessness scores from week to week; and review assessments from pre- and post-group participation. (Assessment measures are found later in this chapter under Self-Report Measures.) Participants can easily see changes resulting from group therapy that make the therapeutic process a worthwhile one. The use of CBT techniques allied with psychodrama provides a balance between an exploration of emotionally laden situations and a more concrete, data-based, problem-solving process.

Considerations for Group Members

CEGT will likely not be an ideal fit for all individuals seeking treatment. It is important that the director be cognizant of participants' BDI, BAI, and BHS scores to ensure that a client is ready to act as the protagonist. Additionally, the director must be prepared to address any spin-off dramas that occur as a result of the protagonist's psychodrama. Although some resistance from group members can be expected, particularly around ATRs being completed on time or disclosed in the group, this diminishes as trust and cohesion grow (Yalom & Leszcz, 2005). As group members recognize the usefulness of the structured CBT and action techniques, intimacy and spontaneity tend to increase, creating and supporting a safe space for sharing.

Individuals with severe social anxiety may initially find CEGT too demanding and may opt to seek individual therapy prior to joining a group. While their experience may be trying, they will likely benefit from the group interaction and support and will, ultimately, choose to participate as a protagonist.

The following exclusions are recommended, as they could have a dramatic, negative impact on group dynamics and cohesion:

1. Individuals with self-centered and aggressive disorders, who display strong resistance to group work. They tend to lack spontaneity and are rigid in their portrayals of significant others; that is, they either insulate or attempt to dominate others in the group.
2. Individuals with narcissistic, obsessive-compulsive (severe), and antisocial personality disorders, for whom individual therapy is more suitable.
3. Individuals with cluster A personality disorders and impulse control disorders, who have difficulty functioning in a group.

What Should I Expect in CEGT?

General Details

- Group size will be five to ten members.
- Group therapy will include 16 sessions.
- Sessions will last two to three hours.

Session Format

Sessions 1–2: Preparing for Therapy

- Discuss confidentiality in groups.
- Begin creating a safe and secure environment.
- Learn about the basic structure of therapy.
- Receive handouts, and discuss techniques used throughout therapy.

    - Receive ATR and Dysfunctional Thought Record (DTR) forms.
    - Receive a list of cognitive distortions.
    - Receive copies of weekly self-report scales (details follow).
    - Complete an ATR or DTR in session (see Appendix B for blank copies).
    - Take volunteers to share ATRs or DTRs (without moving into action).

Sessions 3–16: CEGT in Action

- Determine links between automatic thoughts, intermediate beliefs, and schemas.

- Discuss ATRs and DTRs completed for homework.
- Choose a protagonist for each session.

   - Complete an ATR, and select a situation to be challenged (acted out) in psychodrama (warm-up).
   - Complete a genogram (warm-up).
   - Choose doubles and antagonists (auxiliaries) (warm-up).
   - Conduct psychodrama during therapy sessions (action).
   - Close down; group members share (sharing).

- Process the dynamics of the group.

   - Assign homework (see Appendix B for blank homework worksheets).

Example Techniques Used in Sessions

CBT Techniques

- Completing ATRs
- Identifying/categorizing schemas and core beliefs

   - *Downward arrow technique:* Helps to understand what the automatic thoughts might mean and identify the core beliefs and schemas.
   - *Case conceptualization:* Helps a person identify various rules, assumptions, beliefs they maintain, and ways to cope. This information will come from the role-playing of both the person's own situations and observing others in the group.
   - *Socratic questioning:* Questions that are used to pursue thought processes for many purposes, including to explore complex ideas, to get to the truth of things, to open up issues and problems, to uncover assumptions, to analyze concepts, to distinguish what we know from what we don't know, to follow out logical implications of thought, and to control the discussion. Using Socratic questioning (rather than direct questioning) allows for deeper processing and for the protagonist (and group members) to better identify core beliefs and schemas impacting behavior. See Table 4.2 for examples of Socratic and non-Socratic questions.

Psychodramatic Techniques

- Identifying the protagonist
- Identifying double(s) and auxiliaries (antagonists) from the group

Table 4.2 Socratic Versus Non-Socratic Questions

Socratic questioning examples

- What evidence do you have to support this idea?
- How strongly do you believe this now?
- On a scale of 0 to 100%, where does your belief fall? Where do other people's beliefs fall?
- How does this thought affect how you feel and act?
- Can you describe experiences when this thought was not completely true?
- If a close friend thought this way, what would you tell him or her?
- If you told a close friend about this thought, what would he or she say?
- When you have felt differently in the past, what would you have said about this thought?
- Are any distortions present in the thought you identified?

Non-Socratic (direct) questioning examples

- Why are you being so hard on yourself?
- You say you are a total loser. Would a total loser have accomplished all the things you did this week?
- I'm sure that others don't see you this way.
- What signs of depression do you notice?
- What is the worst that might happen?

- Using mirroring, interview in role reversal, role reversals, and soliloquy during the action phase
- Using psychodramatic techniques to move the group through the action phase

Case Conceptualization: Addressing Schemas and Core Beliefs

Advancing the situation further, the director will likely conceptualize data that has been presented in the psychodrama. The case conceptualization technique is applied as an ongoing therapeutic tool. This technique collects early childhood data, allowing one to reflect on the way early experiences influence their rules, conditional assumptions, beliefs, and means of coping. It is a good way of introducing the cognitive triad to group members who characterize their situations to reflect themes of loss, emptiness, and failure. Beck (1995) referred to such bias as the negative triad, viewing oneself ("I am worthless"), one's world ("Nothing is fair"), and one's future ("My life will never improve") in a negative manner. That pessimistic view is usually a distortion, and the purpose of designing a case conceptualization is to challenge the client's views of self, the world, and the future. Data for the case conceptualization comes from psychodramatic role-playing of one's own situations and observing those of others. A sample case conceptualization will be demonstrated in the next chapter (Example Cognitive Experiential Group Therapy Session), and a blank case conceptualization form is in Appendix B.

Gathering Additional Data

Genograms

Genograms represent intergenerational family maps. Like the traditional family tree, they depict family members, but they go further to bring the family tree to life. Used as a clinical tool, the genogram gathers, summarizes, and graphically displays family history, including medical, behavioral, social, genetic, and cultural aspects of individuals and the family as a whole (Tomson, 1985). A useful aspect of the genogram is that it is not limited to direct descendants or direct ancestors but may include other important relationships such as friendships and romantic partners. This technique gains a visual image of a family's complete demographic information, including psychiatric and medical history (McGoldrick & Gerson, 2008; Moreno, 1947). GenoPro is a genealogy software package for drawing family trees and is the easiest to learn and to use. The software package is free and can be downloaded at www.genopro.com (Dan Morin, personal communication, February 15, 2008). The genogram's visual presentation illustrates the nature of the relationships according to the protagonist (Figure 4.1).

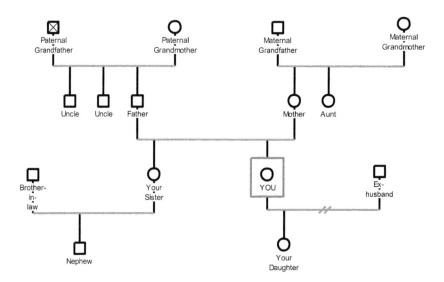

Figure 4.1 Sample Genogram

There are several key aspects that should be included in each genogram. First, a genogram captures the strength of the relationship between the members of the family and significant others, which is not typically shown in a family tree. Family communication both shapes and is shaped by family relationships. Displaying the quality of relationships helps to identify current support networks, difficult interpersonal relationships that may be in need of improvement, and influences on personal development. Specific symbols are used to demonstrate levels of closeness or discord among family members (see Table 4.3).

Second, a genogram reflects the age of each person represented. If any person represented is deceased, the year of death should be indicated. This information is useful in discussing and understanding whether or not the protagonist has dealt with loss and how they deal with grief or trauma. When this information is disclosed, it would be appropriate to ask about how this loss was dealt with and the effect it may have had on the protagonist.

Third, a genogram includes information regarding the health of the protagonist's family members. Typically, both the mental and physical health history of those represented in the genogram are gathered and depicted in the genogram above the names of each family member. This is beneficial for establishing patterns of physical or mental illness within the protagonist's family, highlighting areas that may be a risk factor or stressor that may affect the protagonist's relationship dynamics. Additionally, it can be useful in understanding the way in which the protagonist relates to others during the action phase of psychodrama.

Lastly, when asking the protagonist to list the name and relationship of each person in the genogram, it is important to ask the occupation of the person and where they live. These details can provide further information

Table 4.3 Common Symbols Seen in a Genogram

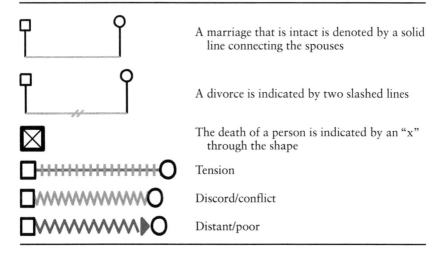

	A marriage that is intact is denoted by a solid line connecting the spouses
	A divorce is indicated by two slashed lines
	The death of a person is indicated by an "x" through the shape
	Tension
	Discord/conflict
	Distant/poor

regarding the relationship between each person in the genogram and the protagonist.

The Genogram Key

Symbols are used throughout the genogram to construct a visual diagram of the family members and other significant relationships (see Table 4.3). Males are typically denoted with a square, females with a circle. A marriage is shown by a line connecting the two spouses. Children are placed below the family line with oldest to youngest captured from left to right. A genogram typically captures at least three generations, as shown in the basic genogram in Figure 4.2 of a protagonist who is the oldest of three children.

Social Atom

A social atom graphically depicts an individual's social network of significant others, groups, and objects that represent issues of importance such as closeness and distance (Figure 4.3). Moreno (1947) viewed the social atom as the smallest group of individuals, pets, objects, events, and groups with whom the person has a significant relationship, whether that relationship is positive or negative. Keep in mind that there is no "standard" format for drawing a social atom and that creativity is pivitol in placing significant relationships in one's social atom.

To construct the social atom, a series of concentric circles are drawn with a dot placed in the center, signifying the person completing the diagram. Each of the circles is drawn at increasing distances from the center dot depicting degrees of closeness. The individual's significant relationships, pets, objects, groups, and important events – including one's job, hobbies, and possessions – are placed in the circles. The social atom

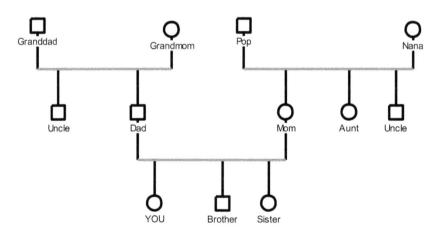

Figure 4.2 Basic Genogram

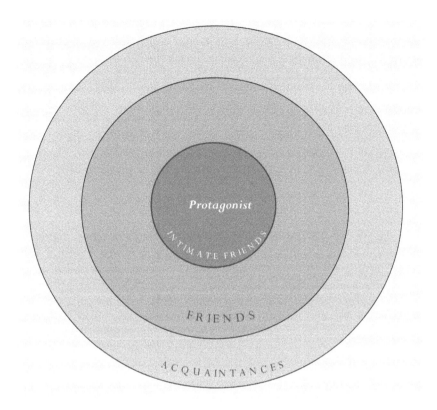

Figure 4.3 Social Atom

Adapted from Moreno, J. L. (1947). Organization of the social atom. *Sociometry, 10*(4).

readily reveals attachments and obstacles at a glance and is useful data for exploring the various struggles in the action format. Appendix B includes a blank social atom worksheet.

Using the Genogram and the Social Atom in CEGT

For the purposes of CEGT, the protagonist's genogram and social atom would be fleshed out on a whiteboard in front of the group after the ATR is completed. Data gathering is the starting point for discussion around family dynamics, relationships, and dysfunctional thought processes about relationships. Once this process is complete, the director will begin to ask the protagonist questions regarding the information described. This opens up the opportunity for the director to engage in discussion and ask follow-up questions about the information provided. Some of this information may be included in the completed diagrams and offers additional insight into the protagonist's background, including conflicts and thought processes related to these conflicts.

For example, if there is a history of mental or physical health disorders or conflict in the family, the director may ask how this affected the protagonist's relationships and his or her personal development. This information may be insightful for the group when moving forward with the psychodrama. To give the auxiliaries information about roles in the psychodrama, the protagonist is often asked to assume the role of members of his or her family or social network. Thus, in placing this information into action, the director utilizes the technique of interview in role reversal and designs scenarios to gather relevant data of the protagonist.

Homework: Alternative Behavior Plan

It is the job of the director and the group members participating in the psychodrama to help develop homework for the protagonist. The goal of homework is to address the core beliefs and schemas through a behavioral strategy. Homework is an essential part of CEGT because it encourages members to practice learned strategies from the psychodrama in their own environment. A sample of a homework plan worksheet is included in the next chapter. A blank copy is also included in Appendix B.

Multicultural Considerations

In our experience, multicultural issues can be addressed in the model utilizing techniques of role interview and surplus reality to present another's point of view. Additionally, during the warm-up, the protagonist has the opportunity to expand on what is important in his or her culture. The genogram, which is usually presented during the warm-up stage, is useful in capturing a picture of family and cultural relationships; combined with the ATR, the group becomes educated and gains insight into the protagonist's values and beliefs. The psychodrama takes place within the cultural context the protagonist defines. When acting out a scene, the protagonist has control over who he or she chooses as auxiliaries and provides, through interview in role reversal, insights into his or her reality. The protagonist can continue providing direction to the auxiliaries as the psychodrama unfolds. This ensures that the psychodrama accurately depicts his or her environment and cultural realities.

Self-Report Measures

Session 1 Only

1. **YSQ-3** (Young Schema Questionnaire): Identifies active schemas a person maintains (Young, 1994).

Session 1 and Session 15 (at the Start and Completion of Group)

1. **TFI** (Therapeutic Factors Inventory): Identifies four factors (dimensions) of group progress (Joyce, MacNair-Semands, Tasca, & Ogrodniczuk, 2011).
2. **GCS-R** (Group Cohesion Scale-Revised): Measures the cohesion in the group (Treadwell, Kumar, & Lavertue, 2002).
3. **CEI-II** (Curiosity and Exploration Inventory): Self-report instrument assessing individual differences in the recognition, pursuit, and integration of novel and challenging experiences and information (Kashdan et al., 2009).
4. **Satisfaction with Life Scale:** Measures satisfaction with people's lives as a whole (Diener, Emmons, Larson, & Griffin, 1985).
5. **The Meaning in Life Questionnaire:** Measures two dimensions of meaning in life: Presence of Meaning (as it is now) and Search for Meaning (Steger, Frazier, Oishi, & Kaler, 2006).
6. **Personal Growth Initiative Scale:** Measures a person's active and intentional involvement in changing and developing as a person (Robitschek et al., 2012).
7. **GRIT Scale:** Measures perseverance and passion for long-term goals (Duckworth, Peterson, Matthews, & Kelly, 2007).
8. **PAS-II** (Personal Attitude Scale II): Measures levels of spontaneity (Keller, Treadwell, & Kumar, 2003).

Weekly

Each week, group members will be asked to complete the following self-report scales and bring these completed measures to the sessions.

1. **BDI-II** (Beck Depression Inventory II): Assesses depressive symptoms (Beck, Steer, & Brown, 1996).
2. **BAI** (Beck Anxiety Inventory): Assesses anxiety-related symptoms (Beck & Steer, 1993).
3. **BHS** (Beck Hopelessness Scale): Measures a person's level of hopelessness (Beck & Steer, 1988).
4. **PHQ-9** (Patient Health Questionnaire): Assesses depressive symptoms (Kroenke & Spitzer, 2002).
5. **Anxiety Inventory:** Assesses a person's level of anxiety (retrieved from Mind Over Mood: www.anxietyanddepressioncenter.com/tests).

Vocabulary

There are several terms (listed in alphabetical order) that will be used throughout CEGT that group members may not initially be familiar with. It will be helpful to read through this list to get a better understanding of the terminology used.

1. **Audience:** comprised of group members.
2. **Automatic Thought Record (ATR):** allows the person completing it to assess a situation and make a balanced decision about the event.
3. **Automatic thoughts:** reflexive thoughts that pop into a person's mind when a situation occurs; expressed thoughts/feelings when a change of mood is experienced.
4. **Auxiliary ego:** portrays actual or imagined roles of people in the client's life; group members who assume the roles of the protagonist's significant others.
5. **Cognitive distortions:** exaggerated and irrational thoughts.
6. **Cognitive double:** (auxiliary ego) expresses the positive thoughts and feelings that are thought but not expressed.
7. **Contained double:** (auxiliary ego) expresses thoughts, feelings, and ideas that are felt but not stated.
8. **Core beliefs:** ways in which a person feels about themselves; three negative core beliefs are helpless, worthless, and unlovable.
9. **Director/facilitator/therapist:** a trained person who helps guide the action; the director is a coproducer of the drama, taking clues from the perceptions of the person seeking help.
10. **Dysfunctional Thought Record (DTR):** another way to self-reflect and improve problem-solving skills after a stressful situation.
11. **Empty chair technique** (also called auxiliary chair technique): represents thoughts, feelings, and ideas toward a significant other who is addressed in the present.
12. **Future projection:** allows the protagonist the freedom to predict and deal with an event or situation in the future; expresses what one would like to have happen; clarifies goals and objectives in the situation.
13. **Interview in role reversal:** assuming the role of the other for the specific purpose of collecting data for that role as well as gathering critical background information; it determines whether a group member is able to take on the role of the person the protagonist had an interaction with.
14. **Minimize/maximize:** minimizing the positive and maximizing the negative aspects of events/people.
15. **Mirror technique:** the protagonist steps out of the scene to observe group members reflecting/mirroring his or her behavior, thoughts, and feelings; one is able to see how he or she appears to others as reflected in the mirror portrayed by group members.
16. **Presentation of self:** talking about "self" to group members; that is, answering what brought the person to the group.
17. **Protagonist:** the person whose life situation is being played out.
18. **Role-playing:** temporarily stepping out of one's own present role to assume the role of another or of oneself at another time.

19. **Role-taking:** assuming a role, one that is not part of one's ordinary life, and being placed in action with a narrow or broad description of how the role is portrayed.
20. **Role reversal:** putting oneself in the shoes or situation of the other person.
21. **Schemas:** a person's pattern of thought; includes ways of organizing new information.
22. **Soliloquy:** unscripted and spontaneous expression of free-floating thoughts, ideas, and feelings as one physically moves in the group environment; it clarifies feelings and thoughts and relieves emotional blocking of content.
23. **Surplus reality:** placing self in an "unreal setting" to gather information on thoughts, feelings, and behavior that have placed the protagonist in a freeze mode.

5 Example Cognitive Experiential Group Therapy Session

Warm-up, Action, and Sharing

The following situation illustrates how to use an Automatic Thought Record (ATR) to identify an automatic thought and then how to use the downward arrow technique to isolate the core belief or schema. During the downward arrow technique, the protagonist will be asked a question repeatedly in order to evoke a response.

A group member, Jane, fills out an ATR and shares it (writes all seven columns on the whiteboard) during the warm-up phase of cognitive psychodrama group therapy. Her scenario is as follows:

The situation began as an argument between Jane (the protagonist) and her roommate, Christine. The situation escalated when Jane's roommate (the double sometimes referred to as the antagonist) yelled and demanded for her to come into the room so they could talk.

Situation	Moods	Automatic Thoughts
I got in an argument with my roommate and she yelled at me and demanded we talk.	Angry (7) Irritated (9) Guilty (7)	What does she want now? I never can help correctly. That bitch! I am always messing something up. **I fail at everything (incompetent). I'll always be alone.**

Moving the protagonist into action: The protagonist, Jane, is asked to select a group member to take on the role of her double. The double's role is to communicate the protagonist's thoughts and feelings that she is having but is unable to express. The double and auxiliary egos also respond to questions asked of the protagonist, and the protagonist verifies or denies whether the statement aligns with her feelings and thought processes. Secondly, the protagonist is asked to select an auxiliary ego from the group to represent her roommate. Using the interview in role reversal, the protagonist takes on the role of her roommate, Christine, and the director interviews her in Christine's role. This is a way of gaining data about how Christine behaves, giving the auxiliary ego an idea of how to play Christine's role.

Possible meanings of automatic thought: To gain a deeper understanding of what automatic thoughts might mean, we use the downward arrow technique to harvest evidence that supports or does not support core beliefs and schemas. The director assists the protagonist in using the downward arrow technique. The downward arrow technique consists of challenging the protagonist by repeatedly asking the question "If that were true, why would it be so upsetting?" This question can also be asked in other ways, such as "If that is true, what does that say about you?" or "What does that statement mean to you?" What is important is that the question is forcing the protagonist to think about what the underlying thought or belief is that is causing these feelings to arise in this situation. The technique can be used during any stage of psychodrama to explore the core beliefs underlying an automatic thought. Initially, the self-sacrificing schema and unlovable core belief emerge:

DIRECTOR: Jane, tell me what you mean when you say that you "never can help correctly."
PROTAGONIST: I am selfish, but I can't let my friends know this.
DIRECTOR: If you are selfish, what does that mean to you?
PROTAGONIST: I'm not sure. I am not fond of myself.
DOUBLE: I put others first. I give into others easily.
AUXILIARY EGO: She never pays attention to me! She doesn't put others first.
DIRECTOR: "Giving in" means what to you?
PROTAGONIST: It triggers my angry side. I get mad at myself!
DOUBLE: I detest myself!
DIRECTOR: And "getting mad at yourself" means what to you?
PROTAGONIST: I can take care of others but not myself.
AUXILIARY EGO: That is such bullshit! You never take care of others.
DIRECTOR: And "not taking care of yourself" means what to you?
PROTAGONIST: I am bound to be alone! I am a selfish loser!

With the assistance of the double and auxiliary ego, we learn about the protagonist's dysfunctional thinking, behavior, and moods and hypothesize alternative behavioral strategies based on her notion of feeling "left out" and thinking "I am always going to be alone." This also pulls out her dependent schema. If the action component is ended at this early stage, it is important to design an alternative behavioral plan (homework).

Alternative Behavior Plan: Jane identified that she pays little attention to herself, activating her self-sacrificing schema and unlovable core belief. Thus, homework may be to design a situation where she will focus on herself. Example behavior plans may include treating herself to a pedicure or massage or selecting a movie or restaurant and inviting a friend to join her. This behavior plan would ideally be created in collaboration with Jane; however, if she is resistant, it may be important to have group members put some pressure on Jane to follow through.

Going Further Through Case Conceptualization

Advancing the situation further, the director will likely conceptualize data that has been presented in the psychodrama. The case conceptualization technique is applied as an ongoing therapeutic tool. This technique collects early childhood data, allowing one to reflect on the way early experiences influence their rules, conditional assumptions, beliefs, and means of coping. It is a good way of introducing the cognitive triad to group members who characterize their situations to reflect themes of loss, emptiness, and failure. Beck (1995) referred to such bias as the negative triad, viewing oneself ("I am worthless"), one's world ("Nothing is fair"), and one's future ("My life will never improve") in a negative manner. That pessimistic view is usually a distortion, and the purpose of designing a case conceptualization is to challenge the client's views of self, the world, and the future. Data for the case conceptualization comes from psychodramatic role-playing of one's own situations and observing those of others. We illustrate next how such data can be gathered in action and how the data can later be used in completing a case conceptualization form. See Table 5.1 for Jane's case conceptualization and Appendix B for a blank copy.

Gathering Additional Data

Jane's Genogram

In Jane's genogram (Figure 5.1), it is noted that there is a history of anxiety in the maternal side of her family. This information may be useful in understanding the way in which Jane relates to others as her psychodrama moves into action. In addition, Jane's paternal grandfather died when she was 18 and leaving for college. When this information is disclosed, it would be appropriate to ask about how this loss was dealt with and the effect it may have had on Jane's life and her transition to college. Jane also reported significant negative relationships with her parents and her roommate, Christine.

Jane's Social Atom

Jane's social atom (Figure 5.2) again shows the degree to which she feels close to others in her life. Jane reported a close relationship with her grandfather, making his death a particularly difficult experience for Jane. Her social atom also shows the discord between herself and her mother and roommate.

Table 5.1 Jane's Case Conceptualization

Childhood Data
Parents separated; depression within the family; attention focused on sister (bipolar disorder); distant relationship with father (forgot to call her on her birthday); mother was self-indulgent and paid minimal attention to her; she is very shy, shuts down, and never felt she was good enough.
Schemas or Core Beliefs Dependent Self-sacrifice Mistrust Abandonment Unlovable
Conditional Assumptions, Rules, and Beliefs If I cling to others, they won't leave me. If I keep anger to myself, others can't get upset with me. If I take care of others, they'll need me/won't leave me. If I show the real me, people will leave me.
Compensatory Strategies I do for others; I put them first. I make sure that others see me in a good mood (smiling). I never let others see the hurt and angry me. I avoid situations that require me to ask for help. I avoid people when I am angry.
Situation Dealing with roommate
Automatic Thought Bitch! She makes me feel responsible for her error! Why do I get angry when I take care of her? I hate myself. I am not important. I am not good enough; I'll never meet others' expectations. I am scared that I am going to be left alone. I have a hard time trusting others.
Meaning of Automatic Thought I give in so that people do not see my real needs. I let everyone think that I am always a caretaker. That makes me unimportant. I am scared that I am going to be alone; I'm paralyzed by that thought. Trusting is difficult; I'll be taken advantage of.
Emotions Sadness, anger
Behavior Withdraws to room Avoids roommate

Using the Genogram and the Social Atom in CEGT

When Jane shares the information that her mother has depression and anxiety, the director may ask if and how Jane was affected by her mother's mental illnesses growing up. This information may be insightful for

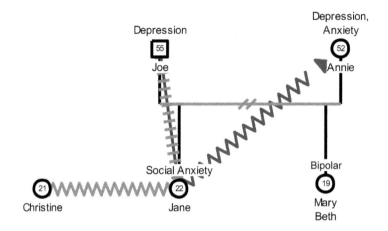

Figure 5.1 Jane's Genogram

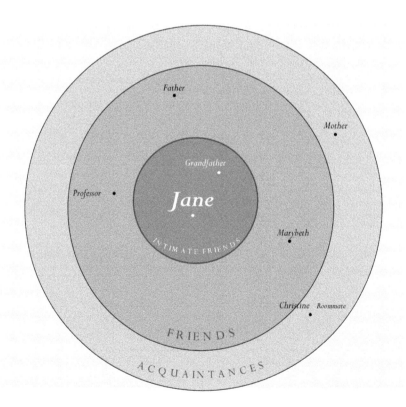

Figure 5.2 Jane's Social Atom

the group when moving forward with Jane's psychodrama. Thus, in placing this information into action, the director utilizes the interview in role reversal technique and designs scenarios to gather relevant data of the protagonist. For Jane's situation, the issue is around her parents and roommate; therefore, the director asks the protagonist to select group members to take on the role of her mother and father. Group members selected are her auxiliary egos.

To give the auxiliaries information about each role, the protagonist is asked to assume the roles of Mother and Father to collect data for auxiliaries to more accurately portray their roles once the psychodrama is in action. Additionally, a double (expressing thoughts and feelings the protagonist is thinking but not saying) is selected by the protagonist from the group members. The protagonist then sets the stage and identifies "needs" that were not being met. In the role-play, the protagonist explores her future with both mother and father. The following short psychodrama transcript gives the director and group members data as to where negative self-image, intermediate beliefs, and schemas were learned. In this transcript, we see Jane take on the roles of Mother and Father to provide information to group members:

DIRECTOR TO JANE IN ROLE OF MOTHER: Tell me about your relationship with Jane.

JANE AS MOTHER: Out of both of my daughters, she is the one that has done well. She does not think we get along well and makes me feel like I'm not worth anything. When her father and I divorced, she withdrew and didn't talk with me. She would always stay in her room and I felt like she blamed me for our split-up. I know she is confused about our separation, but she never asked me about it.

The director then asks Jane to get out of the role of Mother and switch into the role of Father. This usually involves Jane switching to a different chair to assume the new role.

DIRECTOR TO JANE IN ROLE OF FATHER: Tell me about your relationship with Jane.

JANE AS FATHER: Jane is a nice but very quiet girl. She asks how I am doing, and I don't tell her much. And I guess the same goes for me. I don't know much about Jane because she doesn't talk with me. She mentions she is doing OK in college and did say she gets lonely. But I have told her she needs to stop taking care of others.

Data has been generated for the selected auxiliaries. When the auxiliaries feel they have enough information, they take on the roles and the role-play begins as follows:

JANE TALKING TO AUXILIARY MOTHER: I have to let you know that you ignored me for most of my childhood and I missed out on having a mom to help me when my friends were teasing me about my weight. I felt lonely and sad.

DOUBLE: I didn't like you! You let me down.

AUXILIARY MOTHER RESPONDING TO JANE: You could always come to me, Jane. I was around, and you never let me know about being teased. I depended on my mother for financial and emotional help; you should have known that you could do the same.

JANE TALKING TO AUXILIARY FATHER: When you left Mom and me, I felt deserted, lost, and terribly scared. I depended on you, and you left. You never asked about me or how I was doing. I was a mess; kids made fun of me and I had no one to tell.

DOUBLE: I was miserable and never had a father.

AUXILIARY FATHER RESPONDING TO JANE: I left your mother because we were not getting along. I never knew you felt that way because you never showed that side of yourself to me. You always acted as if you were doing well and never complained. You were quiet, but so am I, so I didn't think you were hiding, and, in fact, I depended on you to be good.

We get the general idea that Jane learned the dependent and self-sacrificing role from her parents and experienced emotional inhibition (an additional schema) from both parents. Jane's concern moving forward in this scenario is to focus on the "dependent role" and to explore a new role to counteract and stabilize her.

Next, we move on to the critical point in the drama, which focuses on the "dependent/self-sacrificing role" of the protagonist. The "dependent role" is the role the protagonist knows well, yet we need to explore a counter role, which is a role the protagonist has but has not had the chance to identify. This counter role often is one that does not have opportunity to emerge due to the demanding jobs the dependent role assumes.

DIRECTOR: Jane, there is another part of you that is quiet but wants to emerge. Do you think or feel that role?

JANE: Oh, yes. I don't let that one out because I am always taking care of others.

DOUBLE: I feel lost.

DIRECTOR: Oh . . . and what do you name this role?

JANE: "I don't know role."

She calls this the "I don't know role," reflecting some idea of the role, but this role does not emerge due to her dependent role. To gain access to this undefined role, we have Jane role reverse with the "I don't know role" and talk from that role. Jane is asked if she were to label another role within herself, what name she would give it. In this case, Jane labeled the new role the "confident part" of Jane that is dormant. She agrees that this role needs to emerge.

DIRECTOR: Jane, step into the "I don't know role." In this role, tell us what is inhibiting you.

JANE: Well, this role is awful but the only one I really know. It hides the good part of me!

DOUBLE: I am worthless.

DIRECTOR: Oh . . . tell me, what is it hiding?

JANE: (after struggling) What is being held back is my confident side.

DOUBLE: This is scary. I don't know what to say.

DIRECTOR: I see. Let's move out of this "I don't know role" and move to the "confident role." Tell me about this hidden confident role.

JANE IN CONFIDENT ROLE: I know a lot, and although I am introverted, I have many ideas that I can't express and should.

DOUBLE: It is frightening for me.

DIRECTOR: Let's take the "should" out of the picture for a moment, OK?

JANE: OK, but that is not easy.

DOUBLE: It's never been easy, and I doubt I can do it.

DIRECTOR: Yes, you are correct; it is not easy. Are you open to giving it a chance to emerge?

JANE: OK . . . I'll try.

JANE IN CONFIDENT ROLE: When I need to speak up, I can do it well! When I need to protect myself, I can do it without difficulty. I know I am smart and determined and I can reach goals if I set my mind to it. I have done it before, not often, but I can protect myself.

DOUBLE: I am being judged and need to hide.

To move further, we ask her auxiliary, Christine, to come to the center of the stage. Jane first switches to the role of Christine (role reversal) to give information to the auxiliary in order to portray Christine.

DIRECTOR TO JANE AS CHRISTINE: Tell us about your relationship with Jane.

JANE IN ROLE OF CHRISTINE: I ask Jane to do just about anything for me. She is terrific at getting me out of jams, and I depend on Jane. For example, I locked myself out of my car at 2:00 a.m., and I called Jane to help. She jumped right out of bed and picked me up. Jane is very supportive of me and gives 100% of her time if I ask, which I do often. Many times, especially this past month, I have found myself over my head with commitments I can't keep. I promised to spend time helping Jane around the apartment, but I just don't have the time and Jane is so good at picking up for me. I have not met my obligations to Jane, but she has to understand that I am overextended and cannot help out.

We place the protagonist, Jane, in her comfortable role (dependent role/"I don't know role") and have her interact with Christine. This gives us an idea of how the interaction goes and allows the director to see how powerful the dependent role is.

DEPENDENT JANE: Can you help me out tonight with cleaning the apartment?

DOUBLE: She'll never listen to me.

CHRISTINE: Sorry, dear, but I can't tonight. I have this commitment at work that can't wait, and then I have to meet John after work. Another night, I can help.

DEPENDENT JANE: You know I have asked for help in the apartment, and you are always busy. Do you think you can spare a few minutes this week?

DOUBLE: I'd like to yell at her.

CHRISTINE: Let me look at my schedule for this week. Hmm . . . oh, Lord . . . I can't this week. Work has me down for every night this week plus a huge wedding on Saturday. Sunday, I am going to New Jersey with John for his interview. Monday, I promised my mom to meet her for lunch. This week and part of next week, I am booked.

This is an example of how Jane asks for help and gets turned down and withdraws. The next step is to move the psychodrama further and test out a new role that the protagonist identified, the "confident role." We ask Jane to select a person from the group to portray this confident role. Again, an auxiliary role-player will assume the confident role. It is important to keep in mind that each of these roles is represented by a different chair in order to maintain clear separation of roles.

We bring in an auxiliary to model how this confident role works. We take Jane out of the dependent role and have her sit with the director and watch the interaction between the confident Jane auxiliary and Christine. This technique, called modeling, is when someone else shows the protagonist how he or she would handle the situation. This demonstration models assertiveness and how to respond to a demanding auxiliary:

CONFIDENT AUXILIARY AS JANE: Christine, I have been asking for your help in the apartment for more than two weeks!

CHRISTINE: Yes, I know, and I have been booked solid. I am sorry, but these commitments are mandatory and I can't get out of them.

CONFIDENT AUXILIARY AS JANE: I realize you are busy, and so am I, but the apartment needs our attention. I cannot wait any longer for you. Commitments are something all of us have, and we learn to make room for the commitment we had when we rented the apartment.

CHRISTINE: Oh, of course, Jane, I agree that our apartment needs our attention. But I can't do it right now due to my commitments at work and with John. I am sure we can do something in the future.

CONFIDENT AUXILIARY AS JANE: Again, we are both very busy. We're both students, and we both work as well. Yet our apartment needs our attention now and not next week. If I don't get you to help me this evening or early in the morning, then I will notify our apartment supervisor that I am breaching our contract and leaving at the end of the month. You can stay, but I am leaving.

Jane now sees how another person handles her situation. We bring Jane in again and have her assume the new confident role. Although this confident role is not new, it has hardly been executed by Jane and thus is dormant and unused. Keep in mind that protagonists usually are anxious when relearning a new role, yet it is best to have them try it on for size.

CONFIDENT JANE: Christine, our apartment is a mess and it needs our attention. It needs to be done tonight or tomorrow morning. I know you have commitments, and so do I, but they will have to take second place. Our apartment takes first. It is also a signal of our friendship as roommates, and without your help, you are minimizing and taking advantage of me. I cannot take this any longer.

DOUBLE: Perfect! I expressed my feelings, but it won't last. She'll leave me!

CHRISTINE: Yikes, Jane, you have never been this way before! Is everything OK with you?

CONFIDENT JANE: Absolutely, Christine. I am fine, and we need to clean this place!

DOUBLE: She won't listen. She's going to leave me.

CHRISTINE: OK, I can help a bit tonight for about an hour, then I have to leave for work. Will that work?

CONFIDENT JANE: That is helpful, Christine, but it will take at least two hours to make a dent in this mess. You can call work and tell them you're running late, as you have done before, to make this work for us.

DOUBLE: She is listening, but will it last?

Modeling and role-training are important in learning how to get unstuck from repeated behavioral patterns. Jane assertively addressed her needs, breaking away from the dependent behavior she learned from parents and carried over into her personal life. She has the need to care for others, but going overboard is counterproductive and leads Jane into depression and feelings of hopelessness.

The protagonist chose several individuals to play roles of her double, mother, father, roommate, and confident Jane (auxiliaries), and the group followed her through her drama in a supportive manner. The group gathered the following data from the role-playing and then completed the case conceptualization form (shown in Table 5.1):

1. *Hypothesis formulation.* The protagonist offered her hypothesis about her situation: "If I can always take care of people (self-sacrifice), then I won't ever be alone (dependent)." This was challenged with the following balanced thoughts: "Taking care of others is part of my personality, but taking care of myself in healthy ways will foster love

of self and others." "Being dependent had its benefits in the past, and being assertive is a new role that will take practice."

2. Evidence that does not support her schemas and core beliefs of self-sacrifice, dependence, and unlovability:

- I have an amazing friend (Gina), who lives in Florida; I have been in contact with her for eight years.
- My little sister looks up to me now.
- My dad, who I was estranged from, is now there for me.
- I graduated from college.
- I secured a job as a Therapeutic Support Staff (TSS) worker before I graduated.
- I have more than one professor writing me a letter of recommendation.
- My roommate (Christine) put *us* in her schedule so that our work gets done.
- I am financially responsible.
- I applied to graduate schools to continue my education.

Homework: Alternative Behavior Plan

For Jane, her homework will focus on practicing the new confident role. Thus, situations have to be designed with people in her life where she can rehearse this new role. For homework, the protagonist is asked to identify people in her life with whom she feels varying degrees of comfort being confident/assertive and rate them on a scale from 1 (most comfortable / least anxious) to 10 (least comfortable / most anxious). Once the people are identified, we help Jane make a plan to put her on a schedule to interact with a person rated "3" during the following week in a way that allows her to express herself in the confident role. For example, Jane may be tasked with inviting this person out to dinner or asking this person to provide a ride home from a doctor's appointment. Starting with someone Jane feels somewhat comfortable around will help her gain success and will encourage future, successful interactions.

Additional behavioral experiments for Jane could be focusing on taking care of herself, such as getting a monthly massage, inviting others to dine at her favorite restaurant, or asking other people in her social circle or workplace for help on projects. A sample of a homework plan worksheet, based on Jane's psychodrama, is in Table 5.2. A blank copy is also included in Appendix B.

Jane can then fill in the dates that she completed each task and include additional notes as she works on her homework assignment. She can also use the Fear Hierarchy (see Appendix B) as a way to set up her ranked list of individuals. She will then bring this sheet back to the next group session so that she can share her experience with the group. The group

Table 5.2 Sample Homework Plan for Jane

Homework Task(S):

---

1. Identify people in my life with whom I feel most comfortable / least anxious (rate as 1) to least comfortable / most anxious (rate as 10).
2. Practice the confident role, starting with person(s) with whom I feel somewhat comfortable / not very anxious (rated as 3).

Step(S) To Complete:	*Date Completed:*
1. Create a list of people and rate comfort/anxiety for each.	1. Try to complete list by tomorrow evening (Tuesday).
2. Ask to do something with a person rated as "3." a. Ask out to dinner? b. Ask if he or she could take me to my doctor's appointment?	2. Timing concerns: a. Doctor's appointment is scheduled for Friday morning. b. Could ask out to lunch after or dinner later or on Saturday.

Other People Can Support Me With My Task:

Person:	*Ways To Help:*
1. Casey (double)	1. Could email the list tomorrow night.
2. Michelle (auxiliary role of Christine)	2. Could call to practice for Friday.
3. Erica (confident role)	3. Could follow up over the weekend (before next group) to see how things went. They could call me if they don't hear from me by Saturday morning.

Notes:

---

1. Make note of times during the week that I was in the dependent role.
2. Call group members if I'm having doubts or need a pep talk!

---

members she identified as providing support can also share their experience with helping her with her assignment.

Summary/Review

- **Warm-up:** Select a protagonist from the group and complete the ATR, setting the stage for the psychodrama.

  - Introduce the seven-column ATR, where the protagonist describes a situation, rates their moods, and identifies automatic thoughts and the hot thought(s) (e.g., "I'll always be alone" and "I am incompetent" related to this situation). We then address the next two columns: evidence that supports the hot thought and evidence that does not support the hot thought. Finally, we identify one or more balanced thoughts and have the protagonist re-rate their moods to set the stage for action.

- Review the hot thought(s) that reveal schemas and core beliefs, and, with the protagonist's lead, begin addressing additional situations that have activated the hot thought.
- Complete a genogram in order to gain background information on the protagonist's family of origin as a way to further understand schemas and core beliefs and prepare for action.

- **Action:** Take the core belief/schema and see what the hot thought looks like through psychodrama.

  - The director helps the subject (referred to in psychodrama as the "protagonist") identify a conflict situation to role-play. To assist the protagonist in delving further, the protagonist selects a double from the group who echoes thoughts and feelings the protagonist is thinking and feeling but not expressing.
  - The protagonist selects other players (i.e., "auxiliary egos") in the conflict situation, and, to gain information about these persons, the technique of interview in role reversal (placing the protagonist in the role of a significant other, such as her roommate) is used; the director interviews the protagonist in the role of auxiliary ego (roommate) to accumulate data as to how this person perceives the protagonist.
  - Once all players are introduced to their roles, the director facilitates the psychodrama, encouraging doubles to help the protagonist challenge their hot thoughts and work through the conflict.
  - There are additional psychodramatic techniques that are utilized (to be discussed during sessions as they are used), but the ones listed previously are basic to the psychodramatic model.

- **Sharing:** At the end of the psychodrama, group members discuss the experience, commenting on their experience playing a particular role or on how the situation appeared to them. This section also includes assigning homework to the protagonist to continue working on the new role explored in the session.

Overall Summary

Cognitive experiential group therapy (CEGT) is a type of therapy that combines cognitive behavioral therapy (CBT) and psychodramatic techniques. CEGT is an experiential form of therapy that allows for correction through re-experiencing and dynamic improvement through expression and role rehearsal. With the increasing popularity of CBT techniques, especially those developed by Beck and his colleagues (Beck, 1995; Beck et al., 1979), the treatment has been applied to a wide range of disorders from anxiety and depression to schizophrenia in both individual psycho-therapy and group therapy settings. Although traditional psychodrama is conceptualized in terms of three main techniques – warm-up, action, and sharing – there is no dearth of techniques that may be applied in those three phases (Treadwell et al., 2004). The versatility of psychodrama stems from the variety of techniques that have been borrowed or adapted from various individual and group psychotherapy modalities (Wilson, 2009; Hamamci, 2002, 2006; Baim, 2007).

Review of CBT and Psychodrama

- CBT focuses on the way a person thinks, feels, and behaves.
  - Maladaptive thoughts are examined to uncover underlying schemas, core beliefs, cognitive distortions, and automatic thoughts.
    - Schemas describe a person's pattern of thoughts through underlying, pervasive organizational structures.
    - Core beliefs are ways that a person feels about themselves. There are three negative core beliefs: helpless, worthless, and unlovable.
    - Cognitive distortions are exaggerated and irrational thoughts.
    - Automatic thoughts are reflexive, irrational thoughts that pop into a person's mind when a situation occurs.
    - Automatic Thought Records (ATRs) and Dysfunctional Thought Records (DTRs) allow you to assess thoughts and feelings (schemas and core beliefs) regarding a situation and make a balanced decision about the event.
  - Behavioral interventions are used to challenge negative thoughts through increased social skills and decrease avoidance of feared or anxiety-provoking situations. There are behavioral interventions in which clients may be asked to be a part during their time in cognitive psychodrama group therapy.
- Psychodrama is placing the core belief/schema in action via role-playing in order to gain insight into the protagonist's life.
  - Group members are asked to participate as protagonists and auxiliary egos in order to challenge (through action) the dysfunctional intermediate belief(s) maintaining core beliefs/schemas.
  - There are three stages of a typical psychodrama: warm-up, action, and sharing.
    - Warm-up will include selecting a protagonist, completing an ATR, completing a genogram, identifying a situation, highlighting core beliefs, and setting the stage for action.

- Action will include the protagonist identifying other group members to serve as doubles and auxiliary egos to help work through the chosen situation (complete a psychodrama).
- Sharing will involve group members participating in the psychodrama, providing their thoughts about playing each role. Observers are also able to comment on the psychodrama. Lastly, homework will be assigned to the protagonist to continue working on newly identified roles and/or work toward resolving the situation.

Expectations of CEGT Sessions

- Session structure:

  - Sessions 1 and 2 will consist of learning about the group process and reviewing different scales and forms to be used during time in therapy. Group members will also learn how to complete ATRs to identify hot/automatic thoughts, core beliefs, and schemas.
  - The majority of group sessions will focus on therapeutic techniques discussed previously (warm-up, action, sharing). Group members should familiarize themselves with the techniques and vocabulary that will be used in CEGT that have been discussed briefly in this workbook.

- Group member considerations:

  - Group members will be disclosing sensitive information about themselves, their inner thought processes, and relationships. Thus, group members are asked to be respectful of others in the group. It is expected that all information discussed during group sessions remains confidential; group members will be asked not to discuss other members or their stories outside of group.
  - One of the most important elements of CEGT is that it is data based. The use of CBT techniques coupled with psychodramatic techniques helps provide a balance between an exploration of emotionally laden situations and a more concrete, data-based, problem-solving process. Group members keep track of their dysfunctional thoughts, depression scores, anxiety scores, and helplessness scores from week to week. As a result, they are able to see changes that result from group therapy.

6 Cognitive Experiential Group Therapy for Adolescents

Cognitive experiential group therapy (CEGT) is an effective model for working with teen groups. The model incorporates cognitive behavioral and psychodramatic interventions, allowing group members to identify and modify negative thinking, behavior, and interpersonal patterns while increasing engagement in positive and success-based experiences (Treadwell, Dartnell, Travaglini, Staats, & Devinney, 2016). The environment creates a safe and supportive climate where clients can practice new thinking and behaviors and share their concerns freely with group members (Treadwell et al., 2004).

Initially, all members are assessed using various instruments to establish the nature and severity of presenting issues and to uncover other relevant information. The first one or two sessions are devoted to establishing group norms, explaining CBT and schemas, and describing the session format. The initial didactic sessions are intended to explain the group format as a problem-solving approach for working through various interpersonal, educational, psychological, and health-related conflicts. The sessions include information about the nature of the structured activities so that participants have realistic expectations about how the group will run. Each group member signs informed consent and audiovisual recording consent forms. The audiovisual recordings create an ongoing record of group activities and serve as a source for feedback when needed.

Here's how the model looks with a group of ten teenagers, ranging in age from 13 to 17. In Session 1, the facilitator introduces the Beck Depression Inventory-II (BDI), Beck Anxiety Inventory (BAI), and Beck Hopelessness Scale (BHS) (Beck & Steer, 1988, 1993; Beck et al., 1996) and explains the importance of completing each scale on a weekly basis. These instruments are administered before the start of each session and are stored in personal folders to serve as an ongoing gauge of participants' progress within the group (Treadwell, Kumar, & Wright, 2008). In addition, the GRIT Survey for teenagers is administered, pre- and post-, to assess desire and determination to stick with and carry out a desired goal (Baruch-Feldman, 2017).

In the second or third session, additional data on early maladaptive and dysfunctional schemas and core beliefs are obtained when group members complete the Young Schema Questionnaire (YSQ-3) (Young et al., 2003; Young & Klosko, 1994). A list and the definitions of dysfunctional schemas and core beliefs are given to participants during the initial session (Treadwell et al., 2008).

Each group session in CEGT is divided into three sections typically found in psychodramatic interventions: *warm-up*, *action*, and *sharing* (Moreno, 1934). Many CBT techniques (Beck, 2011) are utilized in the warm-up, including identifying upsetting situations, automatic negative thoughts, and triggered moods; writing balanced thoughts to counter negative automatic thoughts; and recognizing distortions in thinking and imprecise interpretations of difficult situations. The second portion, action, employs psychodramatic techniques such as role-playing, role reversal, and mirroring, which facilitate the examination of various conflicting situations individuals experience within the group context. This enables group members to better understand the nature of negative thoughts triggered by situations and their effects on moods. The last stage, sharing, allows auxiliaries and group members to share their experiences with the protagonist. At this stage, the facilitator may provide additional guidance to the protagonist regarding ways to begin resolving the actual situation in real life. Normally, the protagonist will be asked to complete a homework assignment that will be reviewed at the next session.

Challenging Negative Thoughts

CBT Automatic Thought Records (ATRs) were initially developed for use with adults (Beck et al., 1979). Beck and colleagues (1979) developed the first dysfunctional five-column (CBT) thought record; Padesky (1994) changed the terminology of Beck's Thought Record (e.g., from "rational response" to "balanced and alternative thinking") and expanded the thought record into her seven-column version of the thought record published in *Mind Over Mood* (C. Padesky, personal communication, 2019). De Oliveira (2015) developed the trial-based thought record (TBTR) designed to restructure unhelpful core beliefs with adults. However, little has been done to design a thought record with terminology that reflects that of a teenager between the ages of 13 and 17. Adult thought records have previously been used with teenagers, yet the terminology is not appropriate for this age group.

Emphasis has been focused on designing methods, similar to thought records, for capturing children's expression of thoughts, feelings, and behaviors (see Kendall et al., 1992; Seligman, Reivich, Jaycox, & Gillham, 1995; Friedberg, Friedberg, & Friedberg, 2001) to see how children recognize and make sense of anxious and depressed feelings. It was found by Friedberg, Crosby, Friedberg, Rutter, and Knight (2000) that children may find ATRs to be tedious and uninviting. It was suggested that presenting ATRs in a more simplistic manner would avoid the difficulties children may have making distinctions among thoughts, feelings, and situations. In addition, it would assist children in developing alternate rational responses to their inaccurate thoughts (Friedberg et al., 2000). J. S. Beck (1995) suggested a graduated approach for completing thought records with youth; Creed, Waltman, Frankel, and Williston (2016) designed a thought record for young adults, yet the language does not appear to be suitable for teenagers. Picture-type approaches have been developed in the COPING CAT program (Cognitive Behavioral Therapy for Anxiety in Youth; Kendall, 1994a) and the Preventing Anxiety and Depression in Youth (PANDY; Friedberg et al., 2001) materials for children. It was Kendall et al. (1992), Seligman et al. (1995), and Friedberg et al. (2001) who developed alternatives to the ATRs for use with children, making complex thought-feeling connections more understandable to young children. The advantages of breaking a thought record down into its smaller constituent parts may be most pronounced with younger children. For example, the PANDY materials invite a child to complete the feeling first by drawing a *feeling face* on PANDY and then writing the feeling underneath it. Next, the child completes an intensity rating of the feeling by coloring in the feeling signal (red = intense, yellow = moderately intense, and green = low). Finally, the child fills in a thought bubble or thought cloud to record automatic thoughts (Friedberg et al., 2000).

Exercises from workbooks like PANDY and COPING CAT are geared toward children under age 11, and the language may be found by preteens and teenagers to be demeaning. Thus, a new way to complete a thought record with adolescents – the MAZE worksheet – has been created to provide a thought record with language that the teen population understands. With the MAZE worksheet, a thought record for teenagers, we hope to close the gap between children, teenagers, and adults, modifying the existing ATR and Dysfunctional Thought Record (DTR).

Teenagers' Hierarchy of Needs

- *To be taken seriously.* Teenagers don't feel they are taken seriously. It is hurtful because it is often implied that they are being told that they are not as confident as an adult. Many times, adults frequently perceive that teens' feelings are irrational or invalid.
- *Success.* Teenagers are good at many things but frequently not acknowledged. It may feel great to be the best at practice or in school, yet they need affirmation and reinforcement. Positive feedback goes a long way.
- *Structure.* Teenagers want an orderly and well-disciplined environment at home and at school to feel at ease and ready to learn and thrive.

- *Protection.* Teenagers want to be safeguarded from the dangers of teen culture, when confronted with cliques, teasing, bullying, violence, and drugs.
- *Comfort.* In today's world of intense connectivity, it is easy to feel disconnected, superficial, and alone.
- *Identity.* Teens gain much of their identity from the people they spend time with because these people often reflect similar interests and beliefs. At this stage of development, many teens struggle to figure out who they are or who they want to be.
- *Fitting in, peer acceptance.* Feeling accepted is a primary objective of youth in the high-school context and, for many adolescents, may be more important than academic goals (Crosnoe, 2011; Eccles & Roeser, 2011). Teens need to feel a sense of belonging to feel good about who they are.

Negative Self-Thoughts and Cognitive Distortions

Teenagers may struggle to identify both short- and long-term goals due to negative thinking. Negative self-thoughts (NSTs) are how teenagers explain or justify behavior, or life's outcomes. As a result, teenagers usually interpret negative thoughts as the truth and believe that they are doomed. Some common thought patterns teenagers experience and interpret negatively:

- NSTs happen inside our minds; they are sometimes spoken out loud, but not always: *"I can't do this."*
- NSTs are not always true . . . but sometimes they are: *"People don't like me because I am short."*
- NSTs are exaggerated: *"People never like me."*
- NSTs make us feel bad, hopeless: *"I can't do anything right."*
- NSTs hold us back: *"I am not capable."*
- NSTs lower our self-esteem: *"I am not good enough."*
- NSTs can become a negative mantra that plays over and over in the mind: *"I'm an idiot."*
- NSTs can be comforting because they excuse our mistakes: *"I am so stupid; THAT'S why this (bad thing) happened."*

For teenagers, with confusing thoughts dominating their thinking, the MAZE worksheet is a useful tool, allowing them to see an alternative vision.

Common Thinking Distortions for Teenagers

These negative thought patterns cause teenagers to lose sight of the positives in their world and hinder reasonable thought processing. Thought records help remedy inaccurate thinking patterns. Common thinking distortions, or negative thought patterns, for teenagers include:

1. **All-or-nothing thinking or black-and-white thinking.** After failing one test, for example, thinking, *"I'm obviously a stupid loser."*
2. **Catastrophizing/blowing out of proportion.** Imagining the worst-case scenario, no matter how unlikely in reality. For example: *"My girlfriend broke up with me. No one is ever going to want to go out with me."*
3. **Overgeneralizing.** Making sweeping judgments about ourselves (or others) based on only one or two experiences. Missing one soccer goal may lead a teen to think, *"I never get things right."*
4. **Mind reading.** Believing you know what others are thinking, without any real evidence. For example: *"I know they are talking about me right now. They are thinking about how weird I look."*
5. **Tunnel vision.** Focusing only on the negative without seeing any of the positive or what is going well. For example: *"I can't stop thinking about the question I couldn't answer on the test, even though I got the rest of them correct."*

Distorted thinking leads to many negative experiences for teens:

- Thwarts imagining a different outcome
- Blocks ambition in reaching goals
- Prevents reaching out to create "people" connections
- Limits teens' expression of their emotions
- Overwhelms rational decision-making

The MAZE Worksheet: A Thought Record for Teenagers

In developing the MAZE worksheet, the goal is to simplify the steps to create a thought record in which the language would be more relatable for adolescents. Making CBT user friendly to adolescents involves the integration of existing cognitive behavioral techniques with innovative approaches. According to Friedberg et al. (2000), the challenge for this integration is maintaining theoretical integrity and adhering to the empirically endorsed basic principles within the approach. In order to preserve theoretical integrity and the basic principles of CBT, the MAZE worksheet has changed the wording yet aims to reach the same goal as the previously validated thought records.

When the MAZE worksheet is introduced, it should be taught and completed by the teenager in a group or individual session. This will ensure that the teen understands what each column is asking and the goal of the worksheet. Completing a MAZE worksheet assists teenagers in identifying and challenging dysfunctional thought patterns and creating alternative balanced thoughts which foster healthy choices, improved decision-making skills, and enhanced self-esteem.

When we experience grief (e.g., "I think I lost a friend"), obstacles (such as "I believe I did not make the team"), or apprehension ("I think I failed my SATs"), these beliefs act as filters through which one interprets reality, thus thoughts can easily become negative. Frequently, NSTs can take over and dominate feelings about one's self-worth and life in general. Thought records are one strategy to address negative thinking. Sometimes, they help a person feel better quickly; at other times, it may take longer for the "feel-good factor" to take effect. Thought records take practice, and the rule of thumb is persistence; practicing writing out thought records deters negative thinking. There is great value in learning what teenagers think and care about, and the MAZE tool allows one to notice their moods, thoughts, and feelings. For the most part, many adults think they understand what it is like being a teenager and assume that they understand the issues teenagers are experiencing. They were there once; consequently, they think they understand. These issues may include social relationships, family dynamics, school problems, peer pressure, and many others.

Completing the Teen Thought Record

When completing MAZE worksheets with teen clients, instruct them to turn their attention inward and notice immediate thoughts and feelings. Very often, teen clients feel overwhelmed with themselves and have no idea what they are really thinking or feeling. This process helps them slow down and identify what's going on. Completing a MAZE worksheet in a more reflective state of mind will help clients put their thoughts on trial and gain a more balanced perspective of the situation.

Changing one's thinking is a process that takes time, awareness, and energy. Clients may feel frustrated at first but, with patience, will gain clarity in examining their thoughts and feelings.

Following is an example of a completed Teen Thought Record. A blank copy of the Teen Thought Record is provided in Appendix B for personal use.

THE MAZE WORKSHEET: A THOUGHT RECORD FOR TEENAGERS

Capturing Your Thoughts

1. Explain a recent situation that caused you to feel upset.

I made a mistake in school.

2. List the emotions you felt immediately following the situation. Rate them on a scale from 0 (not at all) to 10 (very strong).

> Anxious (8)
> Stupid (9)
> Sad (7)

3. What were your immediate thoughts about yourself following the situation? Circle the thought that makes you feel the worst. This is your **"negative self-thought."**

> Something awful is going to happen to me.
> I just want to hide. I should have stayed home.
> Then I would have avoided being stupid.
> I seem to make failure mistakes.
> I can't do anything right.
> *I am stupid. (Incompetent)* ◀━━━ Negative Self-Thought

4. List experiences throughout your life that support your **"negative self-thought."**

> I was scolded for not following student driving rules.
> I failed the first student driving test.
> I was asked to repeat tenth grade.
> I used my pen in filling out a test and was reprimanded for not following instructions.
> **It stated,** "Use pencil."
> I tried out for the soccer team and was cut from the team.

5. List experiences throughout your life that **do not** support your **"negative self-thought."**

> I passed the student driving test with a score of 100%.
> I am an assistant for the school's driving instructor.
> I applied to caddy at the golf club and was accepted.
> I was told by the caddy master that golfers thought I was very capable and invited me to travel with the golf pro to a golf tournament.

6. Is there anything helpful about your **"negative self-thought"**? (optional)

```
┌─────────────────────────────────────────────────────────┐
│                                                           │
│                                                           │
│                                                           │
│                                                           │
└─────────────────────────────────────────────────────────┘
```

7. Use an experience from #4 and #5 to create a "balanced thought," and rate how much you believe this thought on a scale of 0 (not at all) to 10 (very strong).

    A balanced thought may look something like this: Even though I'm struggling to fit in at my new school, I met some people at soccer tryouts and they asked me to hang out.

    Belief 7

> Even though I was "cut" from the soccer team, I was selected to travel with the golf pro to caddy for him at a tournament.
> Although I failed my first student driving test, I am now a student assistant to the instructor of driving safety at my high school.

8. Re-rate the emotions listed in #2. Add and rate any new emotions.

> Anxious (2)
> Stupid (2)
> Sad (1)

Cognitive Experiential Group Therapy: Adolescent Case

The following case study presents a teenager struggling to fit in at her new school and neighborhood. Utilizing a specific format with clear expectations of behavior and outcome promotes a better sense of the group and enables the sessions to be more fruitful. The group members are all experiencing some level of depression and/or anxiety. Academic difficulties are common problems among the group members due to a lack of motivation and/or worry about fitting in. The members include Josh, 15, who was recently cut from the soccer team; Brittni, 13, whose grandmother just passed away; Becky, 16, whose parents recently got divorced, causing her to move from her home and school; Jan, 17, who worries about being able to afford to go away to college; both Lauren, 15, and Dak, 13, who have no close friends; Brian, 16, and Jane, 14, who are both failing classes due to problems at home; and Tyler, 17, and Jenny, 13, who both have social anxiety. Tyler is afraid of graduating from high school and moving on to an unfamiliar environment; Jenny is new to the school and doesn't know how to navigate new social relationships.

In this particular session, Becky emerges as the protagonist, and other members of the group serve as auxiliaries and the audience. Becky is a 16-year-old girl who recently moved to a new school. She was eager to make friends and was feeling very down that she hadn't made any connections yet. She joined a therapy group for teens who are dealing with depression and anxiety.

A case conceptualization is presented and applied as an ongoing therapeutic tool. After three or four sessions, the therapist explains and teaches the main ideas behind the technique and asks group members to complete the case conceptualization form on an ongoing basis as the group progresses. A member discusses his or her completed form with the group on an assigned day. Case conceptualization may help group members reflect on their various rules, conditional assumptions, beliefs, and means of coping. See Figure 6.1 for Becky's conceptualization and Appendix B for a blank copy.

The conceptualization leads to the cognitive triad of negative thoughts, explaining how Becky's thoughts reflect themes of loss, emptiness, and failure, creating a depressive/failure mindset. Typically, this characterization is distorted, making case formulation useful in challenging the teen's view of self, the world, and the future. Presenting it in the group may serve as a warm-up for action and provides structure for the group, ensuring that all members feel heard. The cognitive triad readily reveals thoughts, emotions, and behaviors at a glance and is useful data for exploring the various struggles in the action format. The cognitive triad is best conveyed to group members using a visual representation (Figure 6.2).

Warm-up

In the group, Becky completed the MAZE worksheet on the whiteboard during the warm-up phase of the group session. She told her group a story about an uncomfortable situation that had recently come up. Specifically, she had been invited to a party by a popular girl in her class. Although she is not a drinker, she said that she got drunk and the girl offered to take her home. When she got home, her mom was out and her "new friend" said she would stay with her to make sure she was alright. She passed out, and when she woke up, she realized that all her money and the credit card her mom let her use were missing. After identifying her moods, the facilitator of the group began to lead her through her automatic thoughts. Using the downward arrow technique and repeatedly asking her Socratic questions to evoke the automatic thoughts, the facilitator helped Becky to think about what underlying thoughts or beliefs were causing feelings to arise in this situation. Becky was able to eventually identify her negative self-thought. Her schemas of abandonment and approval-seeking and core beliefs that she was unlovable and helpless emerged as she completed the MAZE worksheet. A portion of Becky's worksheet can be seen in Table 6.1.

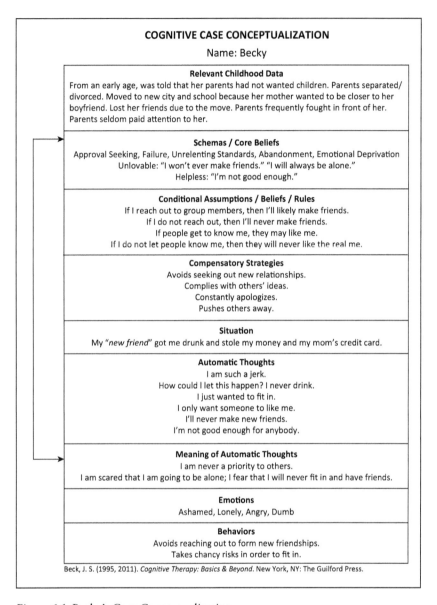

Figure 6.1 Becky's Case Conceptualization

Action

The protagonist, Becky, selected Josh, another group member, to be her double. The role of the double is to communicate thoughts and feelings that the protagonist is having but cannot express. Becky was very

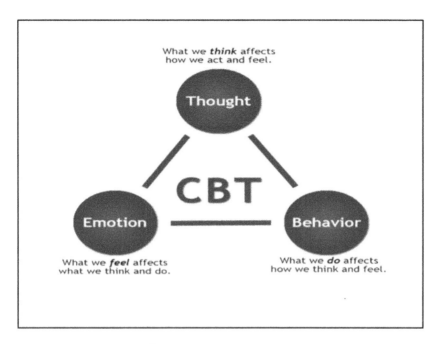

Figure 6.2 Cognitive Triad

Source: Adaptation of Cognitive Triad ©1967 by A. T. Beck

distressed and had trouble moving forward to express her defeated atti-tude. The facilitator used the *soliloquy technique* to help her calm down and express her feelings of rejection. This technique allowed Becky to walk around the room, with her double, freely associating thoughts and feelings. The monologue allowed her inner feelings and thoughts to emerge and gave the facilitator direction to set the stage, allowing Becky to move gradually into the action phase. Becky walked around the room, thinking and talking aloud, and expressing her concerns, discomfort, and hopes. Becky's double, Josh, walked with her, articulating thoughts he felt she was thinking but not expressing. Becky echoed the thoughts that she agreed with and dismissed those that were not on target. The soliloquy technique enabled her to relax, focus, and prepare for the action stage. Additionally, this technique allowed other group members to engage and focus on the upcoming action.

As Becky walked around the room with her double, she realized how her parents' tumultuous marriage and recent divorce, along with the move from her house to a small apartment with her mom, had affected her. She understood that she was constantly looking for acceptance from others and latched on to anyone who seemed to like her. When the facili-tator asked her what she needed to do to address the way she felt, Becky

Table 6.1 Becky's MAZE Worksheet

Capture Your Thoughts

---

1. Explain a recent situation that caused you to feel upset.

   My "new friend" got me drunk and stole my money and my mom's credit card.

2. List the emotions you felt immediately following the situation. Rate them on a scale from 0 (not at all) to 10 (very strong).

   Betrayed (10)
   Stupid   (10)
   Angry   (10)
   Ashamed   (10)
   Lonely   (10)
   Afraid   (10)

3. What were your immediate thoughts about yourself following the situation? Circle the thought that makes you feel the worst. This is your **"negative self-thought."**

   I am such a jerk.
   How could I let this happen?
   I never drink.
   I just wanted to fit in.
   I only want someone to like me.
   My parents fought so much that they didn't even know I was around.
   I'll never have any friends.
   I'm not good enough for anybody. ◀━━━ Negative Self-Thought

4. List experiences throughout your life that support your **"negative self-thought."**

   My parents never wanted kids.
   Even though I cried when they fought, they didn't stop.
   I was always the last kid picked for teams.
   I wanted to stay in the area where we used to live, but my mom wanted to be closer to her boyfriend.
   I don't have any friends at my new school.

5. List experiences throughout your life that **do not** support your **"negative self-thought."**

   I was good enough to be picked to travel with my old school's band.
   My dad came to all my concerts.
   I have two friends that I've had since first grade, and we talk or text every week.

6. Is there anything helpful about your **"negative self-thought"**? (optional)

7. Use an experience from #4 and #5 to create a "balanced thought," and rate how much you believe this thought on a scale of 0 to 10 (0 = not at all; 10 = very strong).

   A balanced thought may look something like this: *Even though I'm struggling to fit in at my new school, I met some people at soccer tryouts, and they asked me to hang out.   (Belief = 7)*

   Even though I don't have any friends at my new school yet, I do have two friends from first grade that I talk to or text every week.   6

   Even though I was always the last one picked for teams, I was picked to travel with my old school's band.   8

   Even though my parents never wanted kids, my dad came to all my concerts.   9

   ---

8. Re-rate the emotions listed in #2. Add and rate any new emotions.

Betrayed (10)
Stupid   (8)
Angry   (8)
Ashamed (6)
Lonely   (9)
Afraid   (5)

was confused. After thinking out loud a bit, she recognized that she had no self-confidence and was desperate for social acceptance.

The facilitator asked Becky to select a group member to play one of her long-term friends from her previous home (*auxiliary ego technique*). She chose Brittni to play her friend Chelsea. The facilitator used the *interview in role reversal technique* to help Brittni understand the role of Chelsea. Using this technique, the protagonist assumed the role of Chelsea, and the facilitator interviewed Becky in the role of Chelsea, giving the auxiliary information about the role. Once the interview in role reversal was done, Brittni was prepared to play the role of Chelsea, setting the stage for Becky and Chelsea to start a conversation. Becky told Chelsea how sad she was about not having anything to offer and felt she would never make new friends. She and Chelsea reversed roles many times, attempting to get Becky to recognize her strengths and good qualities, but, even with the assistance of Josh, her double, she couldn't see herself as anything but a flawed person who would never have friends again. The facilitator asked Becky if it might be helpful to explore a role opposite to her perceived "flawed" roles. Becky was interested and receptive to the idea. When the facilitator asked her to identify the roles she currently plays, Becky quickly responded: ugly duckling, nerd, *lost girl*, and perfect student. She admitted that the lost girl is the dominant role she inhabits and that she slips into the *perfect student role* when she feels like the lost girl is swallowing her up. She also realized that the *ugly duckling* and *nerd roles* feed her lost girl and sometimes prevent her from trying to form new friendships. Thinking about her current roles, Becky recognized that she needed to develop a *confident role* to help her see clearly what she has to offer others.

To further explore Becky's roles, we placed chairs in the middle of the room and had Becky sit in each role – *ugly duckling, nerd, lost girl,* and *perfect student* – expressing what she thinks and feels about each role. Her double, Josh, sat with her in each role, expressing thoughts and feelings he imagined she was having but not expressing. Another member of the group, Brian, was chosen as an auxiliary to play the lost girl, and Jan and Lauren acted as the ugly duckling and nerd, respectively. After several tries, Becky, in her confident role, was unable to shut down these powerful roles. Another member of the group, Tyler, was chosen to play the confident role. After seeing him model this role, Becky, with the help of her double, was finally able to shut the negative roles down. The final step in the action phase was to have Becky, using the empty chair technique, address her "new friend" about what she did to her at the party and, afterward, at her house. This technique fosters interpersonal development by asking Becky to imagine that person sitting in the empty chair and confronting her "new friend." She was able, with help from her double, to confidently express her anger about the situation. Furthermore, she told her "new friend" that she was worth more and deserved healthy relationships.

Doubling, modeling, and role-training are crucial in learning how to get unstuck from repeated negative behavioral patterns. Many protagonists are anxious when learning a new role; it is therefore important to support them as they practice it in the group session.

Before the final stages of sharing and assigning homework to the protagonist, the double, all auxiliaries, and Becky were de-roled. This de-roling technique is an important procedure that allows members of the action group to transition from the roles they were assigned to and return to their own identities. Thus, from each role assigned to auxiliaries, they share their sense of being in character and let go of any negative emotions that may have arisen from their participation as an auxiliary.

Sharing

Following the action phase, group members shared and discussed what occurred, commenting on how the situation affected them. As a rule, no advice is to be offered by group members; only sharing from their perspective is offered. Becky took a huge risk, exposing her feelings and inner struggles; hearing group members share similar painful feelings and experiences led to feelings of acceptance, support, and understanding. Sharing is critical for both the protagonist and each of the group members as they process the experience, reflect, and learn from each other. Sharing is a key component in developing and enhancing group cohesion.

Homework: Alternative Behavior Plan

At this stage, assigning homework to the protagonist is essential, as it encourages the continuation of new role development explored in the session. Role development needs practice for habituation to take place and to move the protagonist to feel safe in the new role. It is the job of the facilitator to address the protagonist's core beliefs and schemas with a behavioral strategy that takes the form of homework. Homework is a critical factor in encouraging members to practice learned strategies in their own environment (Beck, 2011).

In Becky's case, practicing the new confident role was crucial. Becky, the group, and the facilitator collaboratively designed situations where she can rehearse this new role in her everyday life. In her case, situations were designed to focus on developing a schedule to reach out to group members to develop healthy relationships, where there is mutual respect and an opportunity to develop lasting friendships. To promote Becky in this new endeavor, she was asked to choose two people in the group to spend time with before the next session. Although initially reluctant to ask anyone, she asked Josh, her double, and Jenny, another member of the group; both enthusiastically agreed.

Summary/Review

Teens have what they believe to be unique needs that are often misunderstood. These needs include the following: to be taken seriously; success; structure; protection; comfort; identity; and acceptance.

Negative self-thoughts (NSTs) often thwart teens' short- and long-term goals. NSTs are how teenagers explain or justify behavior or life's outcomes and cause them to accept NSTs as the truth. The MAZE worksheet is a useful tool, allowing them to see an alternative vision.

CEGT for adolescents looks much like typical CEGT with a few notable exceptions. It consists of the following:

- **Case conceptualization:** Group members, after a few initial sessions, complete and update case conceptualization on a weekly basis.
- **Warm-up:** A protagonist is selected from the group. He or she utilizes the MAZE to identify upsetting situations, automatic negative thoughts, and triggered moods. Hot thoughts that emerge will reveal schemas and core beliefs.
- **Action:** To assist the protagonist in delving further, he or she selects a double from the group who echoes thoughts and feelings the protagonist is thinking and feeling but not expressing; auxiliaries will also be selected, as appropriate. As in CEGT described elsewhere, the director facilitates the psychodrama, encouraging the double to help the protagonist challenge his or her hot thoughts and work through the conflict.
- **Sharing:** Before the final stages of sharing and assigning homework to the protagonist, the double, all auxiliaries, and the protagonist are de-roled. Finally, group members share and discuss what occurred, commenting on their experience playing a particular role or on how the situation affected them. This section also includes assigning homework to the protagonist to continue working on the new role explored in the session.

7 Short-Term Cognitive Experiential Group Therapy for Social Anxiety Disorder

Social anxiety can often contribute to people feeling like they are alone. Automatic thoughts such as "I'm too awkward," "I can't make friends," and "Everyone thinks I'm weird" are hallmarks of social anxiety. The following situations exemplify the social fear; when we are going to speak for the first time in a large crowd or speak in the presence of those whose judgment is important to us, we all often experience distressing and anxious thoughts. These recurring thought patterns and behaviors are linked to physical and emotional indicators of social anxiety; for example, our feet and the palms of our hands probably sweat along with our heartbeat increasing. As a result, we fear that we will be negatively judged by others, and when we think this is true, we cripple ourselves, believing our thoughts and behavior to be peculiar or strange. If this anxiety becomes extreme and disrupts how we present or deliver important ideas, it cripples our presentation skills. Consequently, this severe anxiety leads us to avoid speaking, shut down, and withdraw, hindering interpersonal interactions. We refer to this performance as social anxiety, and this behavior can take many forms; for example:

- A student who does not speak in class for fear of negative evaluation from the teacher or peers.
- A teacher who cannot attend the classroom because of severe anxiety while teaching.
- An employee who cannot work due to the severe anxiety of interactions with his or her colleagues.

These thoughts and situations make it difficult to feel safe or reach out for help. A group therapy format can be helpful to learn that social situations are not as threatening as they seem. This chapter provides an overview of social anxiety disorder and discusses how cognitive experiential group therapy (CEGT) can be used for the treatment of social anxiety disorder.

Social Anxiety Disorder

Social anxiety disorder (SAD), also known as social phobia, is a chronic psychological disorder characterized by persistent fear and avoidance of social situations (American Psychiatric Association [APA], 2013). SAD is persistent anxiety from one or more social or performance situations in which a person is confronted with unfamiliar individuals or is likely to be judged by others. Socially anxious people experience anxiety symptoms out of fear of being negatively evaluated, embarrassed, or humiliated and ultimately rejected by others. The most common situations that evoke anxiety are performing in front of others (e.g., public speaking) and social interactions (e.g., talking with strangers, dating, and meeting unfamiliar people). Also, some people with social anxiety are afraid of situations in which they are observed (e.g., eating or drinking in front of others, going to parties, being at the center of attention, and using public toilets) and, as a result, shut down to avoid feeling judged.

The Difference Between Social Anxiety Disorder and Shyness

Shyness is more a personality trait and emotional state that causes shy people to evaluate themselves negatively, leading to discomfort or avoidance of social situations (Henderson, Zimbardo, & Carducci, 2010). Individuals with SAD experience much greater distress in social settings than someone who is just "shy." To be diagnosed with SAD, an individual must meet full diagnostic criteria, including experiencing significant impairment in occupational, social, or other important areas of functioning (Table 7.1; APA, 2013; Henderson & Zimbardo, 2010).

Prevalence and Characteristics of Social Anxiety Disorder

SAD is the third most common psychological disorder after major depressive disorder and alcohol use disorder, and the most common anxiety disorder with a 13% lifetime prevalence rate (Brook & Schmidt, 2008; Kessler, Petukhova, Sampson, Zaslavsky, & Wittchen, 2012; Kessler et al., 1994). SAD is more common and severe in women (Asher & Aderka, 2018). This disorder often begins in mid teens and may also precede the development of other disorders, most notably major depression, other anxiety disorders, and substance abuse (Beesdo et al., 2007; Burstein, Ameli-Grillon, & Merikangas, 2011; Fehm, Beesdo, Jacobi, & Fiedler, 2008). SAD is also associated with increased unemployment and financial difficulties, lower social and academic functioning, decreased social activities, fewer relationships, and lower quality of life. The burden of social anxiety on individuals, health services, and society can be decreased through appropriate treatments (Patel, Knapp, Henderson, & Baldwin, 2002).

Table 7.1 DSM-5 Diagnostic Criteria of Social Anxiety Disorder (SAD)

Diagnostic criteria for SAD

A. Marked fear or anxiety about one or more social situations in which the individual is exposed to possible scrutiny by others. Examples include social interactions (e.g., having a conversation, meeting unfamiliar people), being observed (e.g., eating or drinking), and performing in front of others (e.g., giving a speech).
B. The individual fears that he or she will act in a way or show anxiety symptoms that will be negatively evaluated (i.e., will be humiliating or embarrassing, will lead to rejection or offend others).
C. The social situations almost provoke fear or anxiety.
D. The social situations are avoided or endured with intense fear or anxiety.
E. The fear or anxiety is out of proportion to the actual threat posed by the social situation and to the sociocultural context.
F. The fear, anxiety, or avoidance is persistent, typically lasting for six months or more.
G. The fear, anxiety, or avoidance causes clinically significant distress or impairment in social, occupational, or other important areas of functioning.
H. The fear, anxiety, or avoidance is not attributable to the physiological effects of a substance (e.g., a drug of abuse, a medication) or another medical condition.
   The fear, anxiety, or avoidance is not better explained by the symptoms of
I. another mental disorder, such as panic disorder, body dysmorphic disorder, or autism spectrum disorder.
   If another medical condition (e.g., Parkinson's disease, obesity, disfigurement
J. from burns or injury) is present, the fear, anxiety, or avoidance is clearly unrelated or is excessive.
   Specify if:

   Performance only: If the fear is restricted to speaking or performing in public.

Note: Adapted from American Psychiatric Association (2013, pp. 202–203).

Etiology

Like other psychiatric disorders, there is no single cause for SAD; this disorder is the result of a combination of genetic and biological influence, temperament, cognitive factors, safety behaviors, social performance deficits, and environmental factors (Spence & Rapee, 2016). It has been found that children, adolescents, and adults whose parents suffered from SAD have a significantly increased risk of experiencing the disorder. In addition to parenting factors, adverse life events and trauma during childhood such as sexual, physical, and emotional abuse and neglect may increase the chances of developing SAD. Additionally, some patients with SAD have a history of experiencing teasing, bullying, rejection, ridicule, or humiliation publicly in the family, at school, or in society. They believe that their experience and embarrassment will happen again and again in the future. In this context, the role of family, school, and peer relationships is very important in the development of SAD. Finally, cultural differences can also affect the way in which this disorder is expressed. For example, in Western countries, the core fear in SAD is being judged negatively by others, whereas in East Asian countries, like Japan, fear of one causing offense to the other is more common. Furthermore, the threshold of determination of SAD is also different among cultures, which affects the prevalence of SAD among different populations, including the severity of SAD and the impact on the quality of life (Spence & Rapee, 2016).

Assessment of Social Anxiety Disorder

The most popular assessment instrument for SAD is the Liebowitz Social Anxiety Scale (LSAS; Liebowitz, 1987). This scale is a 24-item interview that assesses fear and avoidance in 11 social interactions (e.g., talking with people one does not know very well) and 13 performance situations (e.g., returning goods to the store). Respondents are asked to respond to each item using a four-point Likert-type scale based on how much anxiety or fear they feel in the situation (ranging from 0 [*none*] to 3 [*severe*]) and how often they avoid the situation (ranging from 0 [*never*] to 3 [*usually*]). The LSAS has shown good test-retest reliability, internal consistency, and convergent and discriminant validity (Baker, Heinrichs, Kim, & Hofmann, 2002; Heimberg et al., 1999).

Other widely used self-report assessments for SAD in adults include:

* Fear of Negative Evaluation (FNE; Watson & Friend, 1969)
* Brief Fear of Negative Evaluation Scale (BFNE; Rodebaugh et al., 2004; Weeks et al., 2005)
* Social Avoidance and Distress Scale (SADS; Watson & Friend, 1969)
* The Social Phobia Scale (SPS; Mattick & Clarke, 1998)
* Social Interaction Anxiety Scale (SIAS; Mattick & Clarke, 1998)
* The Social Phobia and Anxiety Inventory (SPAI; Beidel, Turner, Stanley, & Dancu, 1989)
* Semi-Structured Clinical Interview for DSM-5 (SCID-5): Module F, Anxiety Disorders (First, Williams, Karg, & Spitzer, 2016)

Treatment of Social Anxiety Disorder

There are several effective psychological treatments for SAD, including cognitive therapy, exposure therapy, social skills training, and CBT (Mayo-Wilson et al., 2014). Several meta-analyses have shown that CBT is the most effective psychotherapy for SAD (Hofmann & Smits, 2008; Mayo-Wilson et al., 2014). Cognitive behavioral group therapy (CBGT), as developed by Heimberg and Becker (2002), is the current gold standard intervention for SAD.

Psychotherapy in a group format is an available and effective intervention for patients with SAD. Group treatment provides a ready-made audience available for practicing social interactions. Group feedback can be an effective way to challenge the patient's distorted self-perception. Within the context of a group, patients can gain directly from the experience of other patients with SAD in the group. Group therapy also has economic benefits; group therapy costs less than individual treatment, facilitates access to treatment for a greater number of individuals, and conserves therapist resources (Hofmann & Otto, 2017). Additionally, Burlingame, Strauss, and Joyce (2013) have demonstrated that there is sufficient data showing that the group therapy modality is as efficient and effective as individual therapy.

CEGT for Social Anxiety Disorder

Developed by Treadwell et al. (2016), cognitive experiential group therapy (CEGT) is a complementary action group model that integrates cognitive behavioral and psychodramatic interventions to allow group members to identify and modify negative automatic thoughts, behavior, and emotions in action. Both CBT and experiential-action models focus on the discovery of cognitive distortions through Socratic questioning. It has been found that the use of certain structured CBT techniques (e.g., the Automatic Thought Record and downward arrow technique) within the context of experiential-action provides additional ways of stimulating the development of self-reflection and problem-solving and mood-regulation skills (Treadwell et al., 2002). Both during the session and in real life, patients learn to identify, examine, and challenge their negative thoughts. This cognitive restructuring enables patients to challenge their negative automatic thoughts and change them in a more realistic and adaptive way (Heimberg & Becker, 2002). During sessions, patients with SAD can use psychodramatic techniques to role-play anxiety-provoking situations and examine the reality of automatic thoughts.

This group experiential psychotherapy has several advantages. In the course of CEGT, patients with SAD can reenact their social trauma, emotional abuse, and adverse life events from childhood and re-experience a negative social interaction from the past by role-playing, which provides a facility to change the patient's beliefs, feelings, and attitudes about the traumatizing situation (Abeditehrani, Dijk, Toghchi, & Arntz, 2020). People with SAD often control the expression of feelings and suppress their emotions to minimize the potential of making social errors and rejection from others (Kashdan & Steger, 2006). They also report a fear of emotional experiencing and more negative beliefs about the consequences of emotional expression (Spokas, Luterek, & Heimberg, 2009). CEGT integrates psychodramatic and cognitive behavioral techniques to support people with SAD to express their suppressed emotions in a safe environment. The catharsis that takes place in CEGT leads to a change in the patient's beliefs, attitudes, and feelings about a situation (Kellerman, 1984). Thus, the balance between experiential-action and CBT techniques in treating SAD allows room to focus on the cognitive, behavioral, and emotional aspects of SAD simultaneously.

It is recommended that the CEGT model offers broad treatment objectives for patients with SAD when integrating experiential-action and CBT techniques. Although CBT also uses role-playing as an exposure to anxiety-provoking situations, the primary goal of these role-plays is to change automatic negative thoughts. CEGT, on the other hand, helps socially anxious patients to reenact anxiety provoking situations to evoke thoughts *and* emotions during the session with support of auxiliaries and the therapist. Thus, catharsis (emotional releasing) as well as cognitive restructuring and exposure take place in CEGT through role-playing and reenactment. In addition, CEGT endorses in vivo exposure as homework between sessions.

Applying CBT Interventions and Techniques to CEGT for SAD

Cognitive restructuring, exposure, and homework assignment are the most frequently used techniques from Heimberg and Becker's CBGT intervention (Coles, Hart, & Heimberg, 2005). In cognitive restructuring, patients with SAD first learn how to identify their negative automatic thoughts and then challenge their negative thoughts to change them to be more realistic and adaptive thoughts both during the session and in real life. During exposure, socially anxious patients learn to stay in feared situations, practice behavioral skills, and test the reality of negative automatic thoughts. Initial homework assignments typically involve thinking about situations that cause anxiety, writing them down on paper, and bringing this information to the group to put into action. Homework assignments are completed between sessions. As group progresses, homework assignments also involve cognitive restructuring and exposure (Heimberg & Becker, 2002).

Applying Psychodramatic Techniques to CEGT for SAD

CEGT utilizes psychodramatic techniques to express thoughts and feelings that are not being expressed. Role-playing assists socially anxious patients to be ready to face uncomfortable social situations and be successful in exposing anxiety-provoking situations. Key psychodramatic techniques used in CEGT include role reversal and the use of a double. Role reversal is an action technique placing the protagonist in a positive, self-confident role and fosters role development where one can evaluate and view self from the perspective of others (Treadwell et al., 2016; Kellerman, 1994; Abeditehrani, Dijk, Neyshabouri, M, & Arntz, 2020). Role reversal helps socially anxious people to see themselves from the audience's perspective. It provides the opportunity to access the real point of view of the other person and experience how it is to be in the role of the audience. Doubling is the psychodramatic technique in which someone selected from the group expresses the protagonist's unheard thoughts, diminishing the less confident role and creating a positive role to foster affirmative thoughts. Doubles identify automatic thoughts and express the protagonist's feelings during role-playing so that the protagonist can become aware of his or her inner experiences (Treadwell et al., 2016). Other action techniques, including empty chair, mirroring, and soliloquy, help the protagonist to clarify inner thoughts that they are feeling but not expressing: empty chair provides an opportunity to express negative feelings as well as positive feelings; the mirroring technique allows patients with SAD to observe themselves through the eyes of the auxiliary ego/double and obtain real feedback from the audience; and soliloquy is a monologue in which patients can express their thoughts and feelings to the audience. By using psycho-dramatic techniques, patients with SAD can practice expressing their suppressed thoughts and feelings to the audience, identifying automatic thoughts, and improving emotional responding in action.

General Guidelines for CEGT for SAD

CEGT Structure

CEGT includes 12 weekly sessions (Table 7.2); the first, second, and last sessions are based on Heimberg and Becker's CBGT proto-col (Heimberg & Becker, 2002), and Sessions 3 to 11 are based on Treadwell et al.'s (2016) CEGT model. Every session lasts two and a half hours and is guided by two clinical psychologists (one male and one female). Ideal group size is six to eight patients (e.g., four men or four women) with SAD; the group will not work well with less than four patients. The therapists should have sufficient experience in the role of therapist, have knowledge of SAD and of how patients with SAD will respond in a group setting, be familiar with the basic principle of group dynamics and the fostering of group cohesion, and be familiar with cognitive behavioral and psychodrama experiential-action treatment.

Patient Population

Inclusion criteria for CEGT for SAD include a SAD diangosis (preferra-bly from the use of a valid assessment such as the LSAS, SCID-5, or other measures discussed previously), an age of between 18 and 65 years, and the ability to read and understand questionnaires administered through-out treatment. Exclusion criteria include comorbid psychotic or bipolar disorder, high suicide risk, antisocial or borderline personality disorder, and a comorbid diagnosis of substance use disorder (most notably, alco-hol dependence).

Table 7.2 Treatment Structure for CEGT for Social Anxiety Disorder

Session(s)	Content
Session 1 (CEGT)	• Introduction
	• Review of group rules
	• Sharing of individual problems and goals
	• Presentation of CEGT model for social anxiety
	• Cognitive restructuring training
	• Homework assignment for Session 1: identifying and recording negative automatic thoughts
	• Review of Session 1 homework assignment
	• Identification of thinking errors in automatic thought
Session 2 (CEGT)	• Disputing automatic thoughts and developing rational responses
	• Homework assignment for Session 2: cognitive restructuring practice
	• Preparation for initiation of role-playing
Sessions 3–11 (CEGT)	• Review of homework assignments
	• Warm-up (forming a band, auxiliary chair, future projection, behind the back technique, the living newspaper, and milling) and selecting a protagonist
	• Action: preparing a stage, selecting the auxiliaries by protagonist, using psychodramatic techniques (role reversal, double, empty chair, mirroring, soliloquy)
	• Sharing
	• Homework assignment for protagonist related to in-session role-playing
Session 12 (CEGT)	• Review of homework assignment
	• Identification of patient's accomplishment and remaining anxiety
	• Setting of further goals for each patient
	• Identification of methods to achieve patient's goals

Assessment

One of the most important elements of CEGT is that it is data driven. Group members keep track of their negative automatic thoughts, depression scores, and social anxiety scores during treatment. Patients complete the LSAS (clinician-administered version) and Beck Depression Inventory (BDI) before and after completion of treatment. Brief Fear of Negative Evaluation (BFNE) is completed before treatment and after each session. Patients are able to see changes that result from group therapy, which makes the therapeutic process a more tractable experience.

Session Content

Prior to the first session, each patient completes an individual treatment orientation interview to familiarize themselves with one of the group therapists, prepares them for group therapy participation outlined in the consent form, and completes the Individualized Fear Hierarchy (see Appendix B; Heimberg & Becker, 2002).

In the **first session**, the therapists explain the group's rules, and patients share their individual problems and goals. Therapists present the treatment structure for CEGT for SAD (see Table 7.3) and train group members on initial cognitive restructuring skills by focusing on identification of automatic thoughts. Therapists introduce automatic thoughts and how automatic thoughts influence emotions and behavior, using an Automatic Thought Record (ATR) as a guide (see Table 7.3 for an example and Appendix B for a blank version). At the end of the first session, the therapists assign homework, which is to complete an ATR for the following week.

During the **second session**, the homework is reviewed, and the therapists use the completed ATRs to identify thinking errors. The therapists again train patients on the use of cognitive restructuring techniques by using Socratic questioning and explaining how to dispute automatic thoughts with rational responses. At the end of the session, the therapists assign homework, which is to complete the Cognitive Restructuring Practice Form (see Appendix B), label thinking errors in identified automatic thoughts, and prepare for initiation of in-session role-playing.

Sessions 3 to 11 of CEGT are divided into three stages: warm-up, action, and sharing, focusing on role-playing feared situations in real life.

WARM-UP STAGE

The warming-up or ice-breaking stage facilitates a safe, supportive, and creative atmosphere for patients at the beginning of every session. In the warm-up stage, the therapists ask patients to do a verbal or nonverbal warm-up practice in four forms: somatic, psychological, social, or through play, in which patients sometimes do physical interaction games until ice breaks (Weiner & Sacks, 1969). Weiner and Sacks (1969) demonstrated some warm-up techniques such as forming a band (playing invisible musical instruments), auxiliary chair (representing feelings and thoughts to a person by using an empty chair), future projection (choosing a specific time in the future and explaining what happens to a person at that time), behind the back technique (sitting with a person's back to other group members while others express their feelings and thoughts about him or her as if he or she is not present and where the person does not answer the group), the living newspaper (acting out an important event of the day as it affected a person), and milling (getting out of their seats, selecting the person to meet, and pretending to be carrying out a conversation).

Sometimes, these warm-up techniques are considered anxiety-provoking situations for socially anxious patients. This is how the action component of group therapy is introduced. As the warm-up progresses, the therapist

Table 7.3 Example of Completed Automatic Thought Record (ATR) Form for SAD

Situation	Moods	Automatic Thoughts	Evidence That Supports The Automatic Thoughts	Evidence That Does Not Support The Automatic Thoughts	Alternative Thoughts	Rates Moods Now
Standing in front of others in the school	Anxious (10) Lonely (9) Sad (8) Angry (7)	I do something stupid. Others laugh at me. Others understand that I am anxious. Others think that I am weird. *Everyone leaves me.*	I cannot understand what I should do. My hands shake in front of others. I always blush when standing in front of others.	I was able to talk in front of my friends in kindergarten. During a spelling bee, I was able to spell a word correctly and was praised by my teacher.	Even though I was anxious, during the spelling bee, I was able to spell a complicated word and received praise. I can do something truly. Even though one person leaves me, it does not mean that I will be alone forever. Even though I do not always understand everything the teacher is explaining, I can ask the teacher to clarify for me.	Anxious (8) Lonely (7) Sad (6) Angry (6)

Note: The purpose of recording automatic thoughts is to identify cognitive distortions, learn how to reframe or restructure thinking, and write a rational response. Adapted from Greenberger, D., & Padesky, C. (1995, 2015). *Mind over mood: Change how you feel by changing the way you think.* New York, NY: The Guilford Press.

follows the interactions, helping to distinguish which group member(s) may be ready for action. The therapist selects the protagonist based on the preparation in the warming-up stage, information revealed during the sharing phase of the previous session, and/or group member volunteers (Kumar & Treadwell, 1986).

Once the protagonist is identified, their complete ATR is reviewed. The protagonist explains each column of the ATR (situation, moods, automatic thoughts, evidence that supports the automatic thought, evidence that does not support the automatic thought, alternative thoughts, and re-rated moods). Then, the therapist reviews the automatic thoughts that reveal schemas or core beliefs and completes a genogram of the protagonist's family of origin to have background information about schemas and core beliefs. This helps the protagonist and other group members prepare for action.

ACTION STAGE

In the action stage, the therapist and the protagonist focus on a problem that gives the therapist direction in how to set the stage for action. The protagonist selects a double from the group who echoes thoughts and feelings that the protagonist is thinking and feeling but not expressing. The protagonist also selects other players (i.e., "auxiliary egos") for the anxiety-provoking situation. These auxiliary egos are important people who play a role in the protagonist's anxiety-provoking situation, such as parents, classmates, or romantic interests. The technique of interview in role reversal is applied to gain information about these people by placing the protagonist in the role of a significant other. The therapist interviews the protagonist in the role of auxiliary ego to achieve data as to how this person perceives the protagonist. Once all players are introduced to their roles, the therapist facilitates the action and encourages doubles to help the protagonist in challenging their automatic thoughts. The therapist utilizes various psychodramatic techniques during the action stage, addressing conflictual issues.

SHARING STAGE

Sharing, or closure, is a time for patients to discuss the experience of acting the scene and to share their feelings and thoughts with the group. The protagonist and other patients share their feelings in the role of the auxiliary ego, double, or the audience about the action and their alternative thoughts and behaviors. Doubles and auxiliaries describe what it felt like in those roles and the role of the protagonist. During the sharing phase, auxiliaries and other group members also share their empathy and experiences with the protagonist. Advice-giving is avoided, as it is viewed as counterproductive to the protagonist. The sharing of ideas helps the protagonist to gain insight into the situation addressed; for example, a new role or a role unexplored. An additional component of this stage, *processing*, follows the sharing portion and allows patients to examine the techniques utilized during the session. This is followed by a discussion from the protagonist, auxiliaries, and audience. During processing, socially anxious members comment on the action and investigate why certain techniques were applied. At the end of the sharing stage, the therapist assigns homework for the protagonist to continue working on the new role explored during the session.

Session 12, the last CEGT session, is divided into two parts. During the first half, the therapists do additional role-playing and cognitive restructuring. During the second half, the therapists review each patient's development during treatment and work on situations that may still be problematic. The therapists ask patients to set a specific goal that they will attempt to accomplish within the next month. At this time, therapists assist patients with setting goals for the future to repeat exposure to anxiety-provoking situations and practice using more rational cognitive and emotional responses.

Example of CEGT Session

After sharing her ATR on the whiteboard, reviewing schemas and core beliefs, and group warm-up techniques in the session, Sarah volunteered to be the protagonist. A therapist asked the protagonist, "What would you like to address in order to reduce feelings of shame?" Sarah described an anxiety-provoking situation regarding her first day of primary school. Her mother escorted her to school, and she was placed in the middle of the line. Her mother did not like this and moved her to the front of the line. Then, the teacher called Sarah to say something in front of others. Sarah reported severe anxiety: she could not think of anything to say; she averted eye contact to avoid being noticed by others; and she experienced sweaty hands, heart palpitations, and shortness of breath. At this point, the therapist asked Sarah to select a member from the group to take on the role of her double. Sarah selected Jane. Also, the therapist asked Sarah to select a group member to represent her mom's role (i.e., auxiliary ego). Sarah selected Maggie to take on her mother's role. Other members of the group played roles of other classmates and the teacher. This set the stage for action.

We started to reenact the situation with other group members by using the technique of interview in role reversal by placing Sarah in the role of her mother to gain information about her mother. The double (Jane) echoed her thoughts and feelings. Maggie, in the role of her mother, moved her to the front of the line. Then, the teacher called Sarah to say something in front of others. When Sarah acted in this situation, she was anxious, and she cried. At this point, the therapist used a role reversal

technique; this time, she (Sarah) took on her mother's role, and the auxiliary ego played the role of Sarah. This situation, *fear of being observed*,
was placed into action with the downward arrow technique again, with
**the protagonist, the double, and auxiliary ego (her mother) responding to
questions with help from the therapist:**

PROTAGONIST: I am afraid to stand and talk in front of others. I am afraid
   of doing or saying something stupid. It would be embarrassing.
THERAPIST: "Doing something stupid" means what to you?
DOUBLE: I'm not sure. They think I am weird.
THERAPIST: "Being weird" means what to you?
DOUBLE: They would not want to be friends with me.
AUXILIARY EGO: She never wants to be observed by others. She is usually
   selecting positions in the back to hide.
THERAPIST: And what will it mean?
PROTAGONIST: Everybody will reject me, and I'm bound to be alone.

   This short interaction gives the therapist and group members the data
about negative self-image and fear of being rejected.

THERAPIST, TO **PROTAGONIST** IN ROLE REVERSAL: Tell me about your relationship with Sarah.
PROTAGONIST IN ROLE REVERSAL: We have a stunning and close relationship.
   Sarah is quiet but relies on me for help. I am always there for Sarah.
PROTAGONIST TALKING TO **AUXILIARY EGO** (MOTHER): I have to let you
   know that you ignored me for most of my childhood and you were
   always busy with your job. I missed out in having a mom to help me
   when my friends were teasing me.
AUXILIARY EGO RESPONDING TO PROTAGONIST: You could always come
   to me, Sarah. I was around, and you never let me know about being
   teased. I was always isolated as a child and felt lonely. I tried to help
   you to be the center of attention in groups and find friends.
THERAPIST: Sarah, my hunch is that there is a role within self that has not
   been explored. Might you know what that role is?
PROTAGONIST: Well, no. I never thought of any other role. I do have a
   strong self-role that is not visible. I talk to it when I am alone or just
   before falling asleep.
THERAPIST: What can we call that strong self-role?
PROTAGONIST: I am not sure.
DOUBLE: I call it my confident role.
THERAPIST: Your double feels that it is your confident role. Do you agree?
PROTAGONIST: That will work. I like that.

   We get the general idea that Sarah learned the feared role from her
mom and experienced isolation in her young years. With the assistance of
the double and auxiliary ego, we learn about the protagonist's negative

automatic thoughts, behavior, and mood and hypothesize alternative thoughts and behavioral strategies based on her notion of feeling "left out and thinking I am always going to be alone." This is an example of how Sarah asks for help, gets turned down, and withdraws. The next step is to move the psychodrama further and test out a new role the protagonist identified, the "confident role." We asked Sarah to select a person from the group to portray this **confident role**. Again, an auxiliary role-player assumed the confident role. Sarah selected Maryam to portray the confident role. We brought in an auxiliary to model how this confident role works.

PROTAGONIST: I am afraid to stand and say something in front of others. I am afraid of doing or saying something stupid.

CONFIDENT ROLE: Do you know for certain that you will do something stupid?

PROTAGONIST: No, I am not sure, but it is probable.

CONFIDENT ROLE: Have you been in any embarrassing situations before?

PROTAGONIST: Of course, yes.

CONFIDENT ROLE: How many times?

PROTAGONIST: Many times.

CONFIDENT ROLE: And did you say or do something stupid in those situations?

PROTAGONIST: I do not remember. Maybe one or two times.

CONFIDENT ROLE: When you used these numbers, the chance that you do or say something stupid will be very low. This is not completely impossible, but what does happen if it really does occur?

PROTAGONIST: What do you mean?

CONFIDENT ROLE: My point is that even if you say or do something stupid, even if everyone notices, it will not be a catastrophe. You will be embarrassed, just like others have been embarrassed. If you stand in front of others and make eye contact, you can see that not all of them are focused on you, and everyone is busy with his or her work.

PROTAGONIST: I can try it this time without withdrawing and make the most of my "confident role."

Suggested homework assigment for next session: stand in front of others and make eye contact with the group, speak loudly, and replace the negative automatic thoughts with more rational thoughts.

During the sharing stage, Sarah talked about her feelings and thoughts and revealed how anxious she felt during her psychodrama. During this stage, different auxiliaries and other group members shared their empathy and experiences with the protagonist, focusing on feelings of being left out and rejection. Sarah did not talk about feeling left out or alone until this session. She was awed by being in her mother's role and was able to grasp how Mom was thinking. In her words, "When I played my mother's role, I understood that she wanted to help me overcome my anxiety. She did not want to bother me. When I was in her place, I realized I was only doing it to help my child." At the end of the session, the therapist assigned homework for Sarah: to engage in exposure exercises and utilize cognitive restructuring before, during, and after exposure.

Patient Responses

Patients with SAD engaging in CEGT have found this model to be a safe way to expose themselves to their fear of social situations with the support of group members. They shared their experience every week, and they could put themselves in others' shoes in these sessions. Patients reported that reenacting traumatic childhood experiences, expressing their feelings, and acting spontaneously in the CEGT sessions helped them to expose themselves to anxiety-provoking social situations in their real lives. For instance, one patient stated:

> I wanted to thank you; with your support, expertise, and assistance, I could overcome many obstacles in my life, and now I can expose myself to many situations that I could not do before. These sessions were more useful to me than individual psychotherapy sessions which I have attended before, especially since we were doing everything in action. It was the first time that I could express my feelings about my childhood trauma by role-playing in a safe and supportive atmosphere. I can easily express my thoughts and feelings, I am more comfortable going out in public, and I am starting to talk and be less concerned about the judgment of others that I could not do before. I do not feel embarrassed and tense in this group and feel more comfortable than before. I danced at my wedding ceremony as much as I wanted, and I was not at all worried about the judgment of the others and really enjoyed my celebration.

Summary/Review

Group treatment for SAD is an effective method, as it provides a ready-made audience for exposing patients to anxiety situations and working through the underlying negative thoughts and feelings in a safe space. CEGT enriches traditional group-based CBT for SAD interventions by allowing experiential techniques to enhance the change process. The use of CBT techniques allied with psychodrama/experiential-action helps provide a balance between exploration of emotionally laden situations and a more concrete, data-based, problem-solving process. In this treatment, patients with SAD have the possibility to act out feared situations freely in the presence of peers, whether the situation is something from past, happening currently, is likely to occur in the future, or is a fabricated feared situation. In doing so, they are exposing themselves to their fears in a safe environment, reducing the worry around negative judgment. Utilizing the CEGT model provides a chance to reenact these traumatic situations by role-playing and they review how the role of fear impacts them in threatening situations and replaces a role (opposite of fear) that has positive results in action. Catharsis occurs in the cognitive experiential group model and helps patients reinterpret an event in a different, less negative way and gain insight to decrease social anxiety.

References

Abeditehrani, H., Dijk, C., Toghchi, MS, & Arntz, A. (2020). Integrating Cognitive Behavioral Group Therapy and Psychodrama for Social Anxiety Disorder: An Intervention Description and an Uncontrolled Pilot Trial. *Clinical Psychology in Europe, 2*(1), 1–21. https://doi.org/10.32872/cpe.v2i1.2693

Abeditehrani, H., Dijk, C., Neyshabouri, M. D., & Arntz, A. (2020). Beneficial Effects of Role Reversal in Comparison to role-playing on negative cognitions about Other's Judgments for Social Anxiety Disorder. *Journal of Behavior Therapy and Experimental Psychiatry,* https://doi.org/10.1016/j.jbtep.2020.101599

American Psychiatric Association (APA). (2013). *Statistical manual of mental disorders* (5th ed.). Washington, DC: American Psychiatric Association.

Asher, M., & Aderka, I. M. (2018). Gender differences in social anxiety disorder. *Journal of Clinical Psychology, 74*(10), 1730–1741. doi:10.1002/jclp.22624

Association for Behavioral and Cognitive Therapies (ABCT). (2008). What's in a name (BT, CT, REBT, DBT, ACT, etc.)? *ABCT Website.* Retrieved March 18, 2008, from www.aabt.org/What%20are/What%20Are%20Behavioral%20and%20Cognitive%20Therapies.html

Baim, C. (2007). Are you a cognitive psychodramatist? *British Journal of Psychodrama and Sociodrama, 22*(2), 23–31.

Baker, S. L., Heinrichs, N., Kim, H. J., & Hofmann, S. G. (2002). The Liebowitz Social Anxiety Scale as a self-report instrument: A preliminary psychometric analysis. *Behaviour Research and Therapy, 40*(6), 701–715. doi:10.1016/S0005-7967(01)00060-2

Baruch-Feldman, C. (2017). *The grit guide for teens: A workbook to help you build perseverance, self-control & a growth mindset.* Oakland, CA: Instant Help Books and New Harbinger Publications.

Beck, A. T. (1967). *Depression: Clinical, experimental, and theoretical aspects.* New York: Hoeber. Republished as *Depression: Causes and treatment.* Philadelphia: University of Pennsylvania Press.

Beck, A. T. (1991). Cognitive therapy as the integrative therapy. *Journal of Psychotherapy Integration, 1*(3), 191–198.

Beck, A. T., Rush, A. J., Shaw, B. F., & Emery, G. (1979). *Cognitive therapy of depression.* New York, NY: The Guilford Press.

Beck, A. T., & Steer, R. A. (1988). *Beck hopelessness scale.* San Antonio, TX: The Psychological Corporation.

Beck, A. T., & Steer, R. A. (1993). *BAI: Beck Anxiety Inventory manual*. San Antonio, TX: The Psychological Corporation.

Beck, A. T., Steer, R. A., & Brown, G. K. (1996). *Beck Depression Inventory-II manual*. San Antonio, TX: The Psychological Corporation.

Beck, J. S. (1995). *Cognitive therapy: Basics and beyond*. New York, NY: The Guilford Press.

Beck, J. S. (2011). *Cognitive behavioral therapy: Basics and beyond* (2nd ed.). New York, NY: The Guilford Press.

Beck, J. S. (2020). *Cognitive behavioral therapy: Basics and beyond* (3rd ed.). New York: The Guilford Press.

Beesdo, K., Bittner, A., Pine, D. S., Stein, M. B., Höfler, M., Lieb, R., & Wittchen, H. U. (2007). Incidence of social anxiety disorder and the consistent risk for secondary depression in the first three decades of life. *Archives of General Psychiatry, 64*(8), 903–912. doi:10.1001/archpsyc.64.8.903

Beidel, D. C., Turner, S. M., Stanley, M. A., & Dancu, C. V. (1989). The social phobia and anxiety inventory: Concurrent and external validity. *Behavior Therapy, 20*(3), 417–427. doi:10.1016/S0005-7894(89)80060-7

Blatner, A. (1996). *Acting-in: Practical applications of psychodramatic methods* (3rd ed.). New York: Springer Publishing Company, Inc.

Blatner, A. (2000). *Foundations of psychodrama* (4th ed.). New York: Springer Publishing Company, Inc.

Blatner, A., & Cukier, R. (2007). Moreno's basic concepts. In B. Clark, J. Burmeister, & M. Maciel (Eds.), *Psychodrama: Advances in theory and practice*. London: Routledge. doi:10.4324/9780203961100

Boury, M., Treadwell, T., & Kumar, V. K. (2001). Integrating psychodrama and cognitive therapy: An exploratory study. *International Journal of Action Methods: Psychodrama, Skill Training, and Role Playing, 54*(1), 13–25.

Brook, C. A., & Schmidt, L. A. (2008). Social anxiety disorder: A review of environmental risk factors. *Neuropsychiatric Disease and Treatment, 4*(1), 123–143.

Burlingame, G., Strauss, B., & Joyce, A. (2013). Change mechanisms and effectiveness of small group treatments. In M. J. Lambert (Ed.), *Bergin & Garfield's handbook of psychotherapy and behavior change* (6th ed., pp. 640–689). New York: Wiley & Sons.

Burstein, M., Ameli-Grillon, L., & Merikangas, K. R. (2011). Shyness versus social phobia in US youth. *Pediatrics, 128*(5), 917–925. doi:10.1542/peds.2011-1434

Coles, M. E., Hart, T. A., & Heimberg, R. G. (2005). Cognitive-behavioral group treatment for social phobia. In W. R. Crozier & L. E. Alden (Eds.), *The essential handbook of social anxiety for clinicians* (pp. 265–286). Hoboken, NJ: John Wiley & Sons, Inc.

Creed, T., Waltman, S., Frankel, S., & Williston, M. (2016). School-based behavioral therapy: Current status and alternative approaches. *Current Psychiatry Review, 12*(1).

Crosnoe, R. (2011). *Fitting in, standing out: Navigating the social challenges of high school to get an education*. New York, NY: Cambridge University Press.

De Oliveira, I. R. (2015). *Trial-based cognitive therapy: A manual for clinicians*. New York: Routledge.

Diener, E., Emmons, R. A., Larson, R. J., & Griffin, S. (1985). The satisfaction with life scale. *Journal of Personality Assessment, 49*, 71–75.

Duckworth, A. L., Peterson, C., Matthews, M. D., & Kelly, D. R. (2007). Grit: Perseverance and passion for long-term goals. *Journal of Personality and Social Psychology, 9*, 1087–1101.

Eccles, J. S., & Roeser, R. W. (2011). Schools as developmental contexts during adolescence. *Journal of Research on Adolescence, 21*, 225–241.

Fehm, L., Beesdo, K., Jacobi, F., & Fiedler, A. (2008). Social anxiety disorder above and below the diagnostic threshold: Prevalence, comorbidity and impairment in the general population. *Social Psychiatry and Psychiatric Epidemiology, 43*(4), 257–265. doi:10.1007/s00127-007-0299-4

First, M. B., Williams, J. B. W., Karg, R. S., & Spitzer, R. L. (2016). *Structured clinical interview for DSM-5 disorders, clinician version (SCID-5-CV).* Arlington, VA: American Psychiatric Association.

Friedberg, R. D., Crosby, L. E., Friedberg, B. A., Rutter, J. G., & Knight, R. (2000). Making cognitive behavioral therapy user-friendly to children. *Cognitive and Behavioral Practice, 6*, 189–200.

Friedberg, R. D., Friedberg, B. A., & Friedberg, R. J. (2001). *Therapeutic exercises for children: Guided self-discovery using cognitive-behavioral techniques.* Sarasota, FL: Professional Resource Exchange.

Fong, J. (2007). Psychodrama as a preventative measure: Teenage girls confronting violence. *Journal of Group Psychotherapy, Psychodrama, and Sociometry, 59*(3), 99–108.

GenoPro. Retrieved from www.genopro.com/

Greenberger, D., & Padesky, C. (1995). *Mind over mood: Change how you feel by changing the way you think.* New York, NY: The Guilford Press.

Greenberger, D., & Padesky, C. (2015). *Mind over mood: Change how you feel by changing the way you think* (2nd ed.). New York, NY: The Guilford Press.

Hamamci, Z. (2002). The effect of integrating psychodrama and cognitive behaviour therapy on reducing cognitive distortions in interpersonal relationships. *Journal of Group Psychotherapy, Psychodrama & Sociometry*, Spring, 3–14.

Hamamci, Z. (2006). Integrating psychodrama and cognitive behavioural therapy to treat moderate depression. *The Arts in Psychotherapy, 33*, 199–207.

Heimberg, R. G., & Becker, R. E. (2002). *Cognitive-behavioral group therapy for social phobia: Basic mechanisms and clinical strategies.* New York, NY: The Guilford Press.

Heimberg, R. G., Horner, K. J., Juster, H. R., Safren, S. A., Brown, E. J., Schneier, F. R., & Liebowitz, M. R. (1999). Psychometric properties of the Liebowitz Social Anxiety Scale. *Psychological Medicine, 29*(1), 199–212.

Henderson, L., & Zimbardo, P. (2010). Shyness, social anxiety, and social anxiety disorder. In S. Hofmann & P. DiBartolo (Eds.), *Social anxiety, second edition: Clinical, developmental, and social perspectives* (pp. 65–92). Cambridge, MA: Academic Press. doi:10.1016/B978-0-12-375096-9.00003-1

Henderson, L., Zimbardo, P., & Carducci, B. (2010). Shyness. *The Corsini Encyclopedia of Psychology*, 1–3. doi:10.1002/9780470479216.corpsy0870

Hofmann, S. G., & Otto, M. W. (2017). *Cognitive behavioral therapy for social anxiety disorder: Evidence-based and disorder specific treatment techniques.* New York: Routledge.

Hofmann, S. G., & Smits, J. A. (2008). Cognitive-behavioral therapy for adult anxiety disorders: A meta-analysis of randomized placebo-controlled trials. *The Journal of Clinical Psychiatry, 69*(4), 621–627.

Hope, D. A., Heimberg, R. G., & Juster, H. A. (2000). *Managing social anxiety: A cognitive-behavioral therapy approach client workbook*. New York: Oxford University Press.

Joyce, A. S., MacNair-Semands, R., Tasca, G. A., & Ogrodniczuk, J. S. (2011). Factor structure and validity of the Therapeutic Factors Inventory: Short form. *Group Dynamics, 15*(3), 201–219.

Karp, M., Holmes, P., & Tauvon, K. B. (Eds.). (2005). *The handbook of psychodrama*. London: Taylor & Francis, Routledge.

Kashdan, T. B., Gallagher, M. W., Silvia, P. J., Winterstein, B. P., Breen, W. E., Terhar, D., & Steger, M. F. (2009). The Curiosity and Exploration Inventory-II: Development, factor structure, and psychometrics. *Journal of Research in Personality, 43*, 987–998.

Kashdan, T. B., & Steger, M. F. (2006). Expanding the topography of social anxiety: An experience-sampling assessment of positive emotions, positive events, and emotion suppression. *Psychological Science, 17*(2), 120–128. doi:10.1111/j.1467-9280.2006.01674.x

Keller, H., Treadwell, T., & Kumar, V. K. (2003). The Personal Attitude Scale-II: A revised measure of spontaneity. *Journal of Group Psychotherapy, Psychodrama, & Sociometry, 55*(1), 35–46.

Kellerman, P. F. (1984). The place of catharsis in psychodrama. *Journal of Group Psychotherapy, Psychodrama and Sociometry, 37*(1), 1–13.

Kellerman, P. F. (1992). *Focus on psychodrama: The therapeutic aspects of psychodrama*. London: Jessica Kingsley Publishers Ltd.

Kellerman, P. F. (1994). Role reversal in psychodrama. In P. Holmes, M. Karp, & M. Watson (Eds.), *Psychodrama since Moreno: Innovations in theory and practice*. London: Routledge.

Kendall, E. C., Chansky, T. E., Kane, M. T., Kim, R. S., Kortlander, E., Ronan, K. R., . . . Siquel, L. (1992). *Anxiety disorders in youth: Cognitive behavioral interventions*. Boston: Allyn & Bacon.

Kendall, P. C. (1994). *The coping cat workbook*. Philadelphia, PA: Temple University.

Kessler, R. C., McGonagle, K. A., Zhao, S., Nelson, C. B., Hughes, M., Eshleman, S., . . . Kendler, K. S. (1994). Lifetime and 12-month prevalence of DSM-III-R psychiatric disorders in the United States: Results from the national comorbidity survey. *Archives of General Psychiatry, 51*(1), 8–19. doi:10.1001/archpsyc.1994.03950010008002

Kessler, R. C., Petukhova, M., Sampson, N. A., Zaslavsky, A. M., & Wittchen, H. U. (2012). Twelve-month and lifetime prevalence and lifetime morbid risk of anxiety and mood disorders in the United States. *International Journal of Methods in Psychiatric Research, 21*(3), 169–184. doi:10.1002/mpr.1359

Kipper, D. A. (1998). Psychodrama and trauma: Implications for future interventions of psychodramatic role-playing modalities. *International Journal of Action Methods, 51*, 113–121.

Kipper, D. A. (2002). The cognitive double: Integrating cognitive and action techniques. *Journal of Group Psychotherapy, Psychodrama & Sociometry, 55*, 93–106. doi:10.3200/JGPP.55.2.93-106

Kroenke, K., & Spitzer, R. L. (2002). The PHQ-9: A new depression and diagnostic severity measure. *Psychiatry Annals, 32*, 509–521.

Kumar, V. K., & Treadwell, T. W. (1986). Identifying a protagonist: Techniques and factors. *Journal of Group Psychotherapy, Psychodrama & Sociometry, 38*(4), 155–164.

Leahy, R. L. (2003). *What is cognitive therapy?* Retrieved March 18, 2008, from www.cognitivetherapynyc.com/default.asp?sid=768

Liebowitz, M. R. (1987). Social phobia. In D. F. Klein (Ed.), *Anxiety* (vol. 22, pp. 141–173). New York: Karger Publishers. doi:10.1159/000414022

Mattick, R. P., & Clarke, J. C. (1998). Development and validation of measures of social phobia scrutiny fear and social interaction anxiety. *Behaviour Research and Therapy, 36*(4), 455–470. doi:10.1016/S0005-7967(97)10031-6

Mayo-Wilson, E., Dias, S., Mavranezouli, I., Kew, K., Clark, D. M., Ades, A. E., & Pilling, S. (2014). Psychological and pharmacological interventions for social anxiety disorder in adults: A systematic review and network meta-analysis. *The Lancet Psychiatry, 1*(5), 368–376. doi:10.1016/S2215-0366(14)70329-3

McGoldrick, M., & Gerson, R. (2008). *Genograms: Assessment and intervention* (3rd ed.). New York: W.W. Norton Publishing Co.

Moreno, J. L. (1934). *Who shall survive? A new approach to the problem of human interrelations.* Washington, DC: Nervous & Mental Disease.

Moreno, J. L. (1947). Organization of the social atom. *Sociometry, 10*(4), 287–293.

Moreno, J. L. (1953). *Who shall survive? Foundations of sociometry, group therapy and sociodrama* (2nd ed., pp. 81–91). New York: Beacon House.

Moreno, J. L. (1972). *Psychodrama* (vol. 1, 4th ed.). New York: Beacon House Press.

Padesky, C. A. (1994). Schema change processes in cognitive therapy. *Clinical Psychology & Psychotherapy, 1*(5), 267–278.

Patel, A., Knapp, M., Henderson, J., & Baldwin, D. (2002). The economic consequences of social phobia. *Journal of Affective Disorders, 68*(2–3), 221–233. doi:10.1016/S0165-0327(00)00323-2

Robitschek, C., Ashton, M. W., Spering, C. C., Geiger, N., Byers, D., Schotts, G. C., & Thoen, M. (2012). Development and psychometric properties of the Personal Growth Initiative Scale-II. *Journal of Counseling Psychology, 59*, 274–287. doi:10.1037/a0027310

Rodebaugh, T. L., Woods, C. M., Thissen, D. M., Heimberg, R. G., Chambless, D. L., & Rapee, R. M. (2004). More information from fewer questions: The factor structure and item properties of the original and Brief Fear of Negative Evaluation Scale. *Psychological Assessment, 16*(2), 169. doi:10.1037/1040-3590.16.2.169

Sarol-Kulka, A. (2004). Jacob Levy Moreno and his theory of creativity and spontaneity. *Psychoterapia, 4*(131).

Schact, M. (2007). Spontaneity-creativity: The psychodramatic concept of change. In B. Clark, J. Burmeister, & M. Maciel (Eds.), *Psychodrama: Advances in theory and practice.* London: Routledge. https://doi.org/10.4324/9780203961100

Seligman, M. E., Reivich, K., Jaycox, L., & Gillham, J. (1995). *The optimistic child.* Boston: Houghton Mifflin.

Shay, J. J. (2017). Contemporary models of group therapy: Where are we today? *International Journal of Group Psychotherapy, 67*, 7–12.

Spence, S. H., & Rapee, R. M. (2016). The etiology of social anxiety disorder: An evidenced-based model. *Behaviour Research and Therapy, 86*, 50–67. doi:10.1016.2016.06.007

Spokas, M., Luterek, J. A., & Heimberg, R. G. (2009). Social anxiety and emotional suppression: The mediating role of beliefs. *Journal of Behavior Therapy and Experimental Psychiatry, 40*(2), 283–291. doi:10.1016/j.jbtep.2008.12.004

Steger, M. F., Frazier, P., Oishi, S., & Kaler, M. (2006). The meaning in life questionnaire: Assessing the presence of and search for meaning in life. *Journal of Counseling Psychology, 53*, 80–93.

Tomson, P. V. (1985). Genograms in general practice. *Journal of the Royal Society of Medicine* (Supplement), *78*(8), 34–39.

Treadwell, T. W., Dartnell, D., Travaglini, L., Staats, M., & Devinney, K. (2016). *Group therapy workbook: Integrating cognitive behavioral therapy with psychodramatic theory and practice.* Parker, CO: Outskirts Publishing.

Treadwell, T. W., & Kumar, V. K. (2002). Introduction to the special issue on cognitive behavioral therapy and psychodrama. *Journal of Group Psychotherapy, Psychodrama and Sociometry, 55*(2–3), 51.

Treadwell, T. W., Kumar, V. K., & Lavertue, N. (2002). The Group Cohesion Scale–Revised: Reliability & validity. *International Journal of Action Methods, 54*(1), 3–12.

Treadwell, T. W., Kumar, V. K., & Wright, J. (2002). Enriching psychodrama via the use of cognitive behavioral therapy techniques. *Journal of Group Psychotherapy, Psychodrama, & Sociometry, 55*, 55–65.

Treadwell, T. W., Kumar, V. K., & Wright, J. (2004). Enriching psychodrama via the use of cognitive behavioral therapy techniques. *Journal of Group Psychotherapy, Psychodrama, & Sociometry, 55*, 55–65.

Treadwell, T. W., Kumar, V. K., & Wright, J. (2008). Group cognitive behavioral model: Integrating cognitive behavioral with psychodramatic theory and techniques. In S. S. Fehr (Ed.), *101 interventions in group therapy.* New York: The Hayworth Press.

Treadwell, T. W., Travaglini, L., Reisch, E., & Kumar, V. K. (2011). The effectiveness of collaborative story building and telling in facilitating group cohesion in a college classroom setting. *International Journal of Group Psychotherapy, 61*(4), 502–517.

Watson, D., & Friend, R. (1969). Measurement of social-evaluative anxiety. *Journal of Consulting and Clinical Psychology, 33*(4), 448. doi:10.1037/h0020196

Weeks, J. W., Heimberg, R. G., Fresco, D. M., Hart, T. A., Turk, C. L., Schneier, F. R., & Liebowitz, M. R. (2005). Empirical validation and psychometric evaluation of the Brief Fear of Negative Evaluation Scale in patients with social anxiety disorder. *Psychological Assessment, 17*(2), 179. doi:10.1037/1040-3590.17.2.179

Weiner, H. B., & Sacks, J. M. (1969). Warm-up and sum-up. *Group Psychotherapy, 22*(1–2), 85–102.

Wilson, J. (2009). An introduction to psychodrama for CBT practitioners. *Journal of the New Zealand College of Clinical Psychologists, 19*, 4–7.

Wilson, J. (2011). Psychodrama and cognitive behavioral therapy: Complementary companions. *The Group Psychologist, 21*(2), 10–17.

Woolfolk, R. (2000). Cognition and emotion in counseling and psychotherapy. *Practical Philosophy, 3*(3), 19–27.

Yalom, I. D., & Leszcz, M. (2005). *The theory and practice of group psychotherapy* (5th ed.). New York, NY: Basic Books.

Young, J. E. (1994). *Cognitive therapy for personality disorders: A schema-focused approach.* Sarasota, FL: Professional Resources Press.

Young, J. E., & Klosko, J. S. (1994). *Reinventing your life.* New York: Plume.

Young, J. E., Klosko, J. S., & Weishaar, M. E. (2003). *Schema therapy: A practitioner's guide.* New York, NY: The Guilford Press.

Appendix A
Cognitive Distortions

Twelve different cognitive distortions are outlined by Beck (2011):

1. *All-or-nothing thinking* (also called black-and-white, polarized, or dichotomous thinking): You view a situation in only two categories instead of on a continuum.

   Example: "If I'm not a total success, I'm a failure."

2. *Catastrophizing* (also called fortune-telling): You predict the future negatively without considering other, more likely outcomes.

   Example: "I'll be so upset; I won't be able to function at all."

3. *Disqualifying or discounting the positive:* You unreasonably tell yourself that positive experiences, deeds, or qualities do not count.

   Example: "I did that project well, but that doesn't mean I'm competent; I just got lucky."

4. *Emotional reasoning:* You think something must be true because you "feel" (actually believe) it so strongly, ignoring or discounting evidence to the contrary.

   Example: "I know I do a lot of things OK at work, but I still feel like I'm a failure."

5. *Labeling:* You put a fixed, global label on yourself or others without considering that the evidence might more reasonably lead to a less disastrous conclusion.

   Example: "I'm a loser. He's no good."

6. *Magnification/minimization:* When you evaluate yourself, another person, or a situation, you unreasonably magnify the negative and/or minimize the positive.

   Example: "Getting a mediocre evaluation proves how inadequate I am. Getting high marks doesn't mean I'm smart."

7. *Mental filter* (also called selective abstraction): You pay undue attention to one negative detail instead of seeing the whole picture.

Example: "Because I got one low rating on my evaluation [which also contained several high ratings], it means I'm doing a lousy job."

8. *Mind reading:* You believe you know what others are thinking, failing to consider other, more likely possibilities.

Example: "He's thinks I don't know the first thing about this project."

9. *Overgeneralization:* You make a sweeping negative conclusion that goes far beyond the current situation.

Example: "[Because I felt uncomfortable at the meeting] I don't have what it takes to make friends."

10. *Personalization:* You believe others are behaving negatively because of you, without considering more plausible explanations for their behavior.

Example: "The repairman was curt to me because I did something wrong."

11. *"Should" and "must" statements* (also called imperatives): You must have a precise, fixed idea of how you or others should behave, and you overestimate how bad it is when these expectations are not met.

Example: "It's terrible that I made a mistake. I should have known the right thing to do."

12. *Tunnel vision:* You only see the negative aspects of a situation.

Example: "My son's teacher can't do anything right. He's critical and insensitive and lousy at teaching."

Appendix B
Blank Worksheets

Automatic Thought Record

Situation	Moods	Automatic Thoughts (Images)	Evidence That Supports The Hot Thought	Evidence That Does Not Support The Hot Thought	Alternative/ Balanced Thoughts	Rate Moods Now
Who were you with? What were you doing? When was it? Where were you?	Describe each mood in one word. Rate intensity of mood (0–100%).	Answer some or all of the following questions: What was going through my mind just before I started to feel this way? What does this say about me? What does this mean about me? My life? My future? What am I afraid might happen? What is the worst thing that could happen if this is true? What does this mean about how the other person or other people feel or think about me? What does this mean about the other person or people in general? What images or memories do I have in this situation?	Circle hot thought in the previous column for which you are looking for evidence. Write factual evidence to support this conclusion. (Try to avoid mind reading and interpretation of facts.)		Write an alternative or balanced thought. Rate how much you believe in each alternative or balanced thought (0–100%).	Copy the feelings from Column 2. Re-rate the intensity of each feeling from 0 to 100% as well as any new records.

Adapted from Greenberger, D., & Padesky, C. (1995, 2015). *Mind over mood: Change how you feel by changing the way you think*. New York, NY: The Guilford Press.

Dysfunctional Thought Record

Date and time	Situation	Automatic thought(s)	Emotion(s)	Adaptive response	Outcome
	What event, stream of thoughts, daydreams, or recollection led to the unpleasant emotion? What (if any) distressing physical sensations did you have?	What thoughts and/or images went through your mind? How much did you believe each one at the time?	What emotion(s) (sad, anxious, angry, etc.) did you feel at the time? How intense (0–100%) was the emotion?	(Optional) What cognitive distortion did you make? Compose a response to the automatic thoughts. How much do you believe each response?	How much do you now believe each automatic thought? What emotion do you feel now? How intense (0–100%) is the emotion? What will you (or did you) do?

Adaptation of Dysfunctional Thought Record © 2011 by Judith Beck, PhD.

Cognitive Conceptualization Diagram

Name_____   Date_____

Relevant childhood data

Schemas / Core Beliefs

Conditional Assumptions / Beliefs / Rules

Compensatory Strategies

Situation

Automatic Thought(s)

Meaning of Automatic Thought(s)

Emotion

Behaviors

Likely Cognitive Distortions

Activity Scheduling and Monitoring Worksheet

Within each time slot, record (1) what you did (brief description), (2) your sense of pleasure for the activity on a 0 (no pleasure) to 10 (maximum pleasure) scale (P = 0–10), and (3) your sense of achievement for the activity (A = 0–10). Example: watching TV, P = 8, A = 2.

WEEK OF: _____

	MONDAY	TUESDAY	WEDNESDAY	THURSDAY	FRIDAY	SATURDAY	SUNDAY
12 a.m.–6 a.m.							
6 a.m.–8 a.m.							
8 a.m.–10 a.m.							
10 a.m.–12 p.m.							
12 p.m.–2 p.m.							
2 p.m.–4 p.m.							
4 p.m.–6 p.m.							
6 p.m.–8 p.m.							
8 p.m.–10 p.m.							
10 p.m.–12 a.m.							

Adapted from *Cognitive Behavioral Therapy Self-Help Resources* (2010), www.getselfhelp.co.uk/freedownloads2.htm.

Goal-Setting Worksheet

Long-Term Goal 1

| |
| |

Steps to Reach Goal 1

| a. |
| b. |
| c. |
| d. |

Long-Term Goal 2

| |
| |

Steps to Reach Goal 2

| a. |
| b. |
| c. |
| d. |

Graded Exposure

GOAL:				
STEP(S)		PRE-STEP DISTRESS (1–10)	IN-THE-MOMENT DISTRESS (1–10)	POST-STEP DISTRESS (1–10)
a.				
b.				
c.				
d.				
e.				
f.				
g.				
h.				

GOAL:				
STEP(S)		PRE-STEP DISTRESS (1–10)	IN-THE-MOMENT DISTRESS (1–10)	Post-Step Distress (1–10)
a.				
b.				
c.				
d.				
e.				
f.				
g.				
h.				

Fear Hierarchy

Directions: Write down all the situations that distress you, then add them to the table in order of how distressing they are. In the last column, rate how distressed each one makes you from 0 (no distress) to 10 (maximum distress).

RANK	FEARED SITUATION	NORMALLY AVOID? (YES/NO)	DISTRESS

Adapted from *Cognitive Behavioral Therapy Self-Help Resources* (2010), www.getselfhelp.co.uk/freedownloads2.htm.

Homework Plan

HOMEWORK TASK(S):

STEP(S) TO COMPLETE: DATE COMPLETED:

OTHER PEOPLE CAN SUPPORT ME WITH MY TASK:

PERSON: WAYS TO HELP:

NOTES:

Social Atom

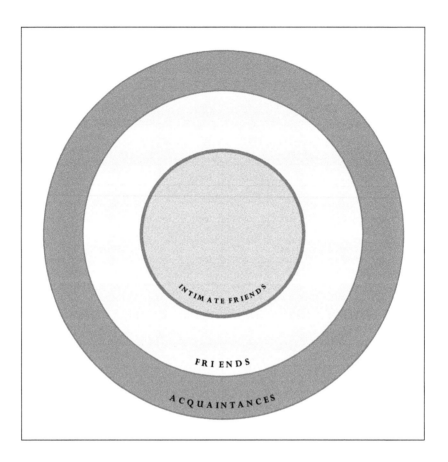

The MAZE Worksheet: A Thought Record for Teenagers

EXPLORING THE
MAZE OF LIFE

One Thought at a Time

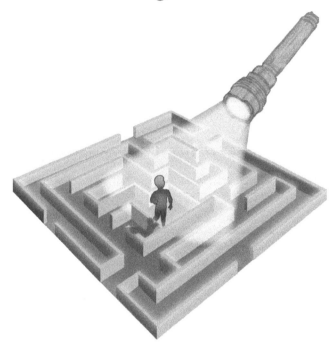

Life is full of extraordinary moments and complex situations that we maneuver through. As you continue through these pages, you will be provided with a variety of tools to help shed light on the pathways of your thoughts, but it will be up to you to decide how to navigate your maze.

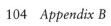

CAPTURE YOUR THOUGHTS
1. Explain a recent situation that caused you to feel upset.
2. List the emotions you felt immediately following the situation. Rate them on a scale from 0 (not at all) to 10 (very strong).
3. What were your immediate thoughts about yourself following the situation? Circle the thought that makes you feel the worst. This is your **"negative self-thought."**
4. List experiences throughout your life that support your **"negative self-thought."**
5. List experiences throughout your life that **do not** support your **"negative self-thought."**
6. Is there anything helpful about your **"negative self-thought"**? (optional)
7. Use an experience from #4 and #5 to create a "balanced thought," and rate how much you believe this thought on a scale of 0 (not at all) to 10 (very strong). *A balanced thought may look something like this: Even though I'm struggling to fit in at my new school, I met some people at soccer tryouts and they asked me to hang out. (Belief = 7)*
8. Re-rate the emotions listed in #2. Add and rate any new emotions.

Adapted from Greenberger, D., & Padesky, C. (1995, 2015). *Mind over mood: Change how you feel by changing the way you think*. New York, NY: The Guilford Press.

Cognitive Restructuring Practice Form

1. Situation:	
2. Automatic thoughts:	3. Thinking errors:

4. Emotions you feel as you think these thoughts (check boxes that apply):

☐ Anxious/nervous   ☐ Frustrated   ☐ Irritated   ☐ Ashamed
☐ Angry   ☐ Sad   ☐ Embarrassed   ☐ Hateful
☐ Other(s): _____

5. Challenges: (Use the disputing questions below or others you prefer. Challenge the most important automatic thoughts you listed above. Be careful to answer the questions raised by the disputing question.)

DISPUTING QUESTIONS: Do I know for certain that _____? Am I 100% sure that _____? What evidence do I have that _____? What is the worst that could happen? How bad is that? Do I have a crystal ball? Is there another explanation for _____? Does _____ have to lead to or equal _____? Is there another point of view? What does _____ mean? Does _____ really mean that I am a(n) _____?

6. Rational response(s):

Appendix C
Certified Training

The fields of cognitive behavioral therapy (CBT) and group psychotherapy and psychodrama have established standards for differentiating those who have fulfilled a recognized course of training. In the mid-1970s, the American Board of Examiners (ABE) in Psychodrama, Sociometry, and Group Psychotherapy was formed and established two levels of proficiency: certified practitioner (CP) and Trainer, Educator, and Practitioner (TEP). Likewise, in October 1996, a group of cognitive therapists met to discuss the merits of creating an organization to educate the public about cognitive therapy and to certify qualified mental health professionals in cognitive therapy. As a result, the Academy of Cognitive Therapy (ACT) was developed as a means to identify and credential mental health professionals who demonstrate competence in cognitive therapy.

Both organizations have established criteria for competence in each specialty. For those interested in pursuing training in psychodrama and CBT, please write or email:

Academy of Cognitive Therapy	American Board of Examiners in Psychodrama, Sociometry, and Group Psychotherapy
245 N. 15th Street, MS 403 17 New College Building Department of Psychiatry Philadelphia, PA 19102	PO Box 15572 Washington, DC 20003-0572
Fax: 215-537-1789 **Email:** info@academyofct.org	**Phone:** 202-483-0514 **Email:** abepsychodrama@yahoo.com
Web: www.academyofct.org/cbt-training-and-consultation	**Web:** www.psychodramacertification.org

Index